Reclaiming Our Health

YALE UNIVERSITY PRESS HEALTH & WELLNESS

A Yale University Press Health & Wellness book is an authoritative, accessible source of information on a health-related topic. It may provide guidance to help you lead a healthy life, examine your treatment options for a specific condition or disease, situate a healthcare issue in the context of your life as a whole, or address questions or concerns that linger after visits to your healthcare provider.

JOSEPH A. ABBOUD, M.D., and SOO KIM ABBOUD, M.D., *No More Joint Pain*

THOMAS E. BROWN, Ph.D., *Attention Deficit Disorder: The Unfocused Mind in Children and Adults*

PATRICK CONLON, *The Essential Hospital Handbook: How to Be an Effective Partner in a Loved One's Care*

RICHARD C. FRANK, M.D., *Fighting Cancer with Knowledge and Hope: A Guide for Patients, Families, and Health Care Providers*

MICHELLE A. GOURDINE, M.D., *Reclaiming Our Health: A Guide to African American Wellness*

MARJORIE GREENFIELD, M.D., *The Working Woman's Pregnancy Book*

RUTH H. GROBSTEIN, M.D., Ph.D., *The Breast Cancer Book: What You Need to Know to Make Informed Decisions*

JAMES W. HICKS, M.D., *Fifty Signs of Mental Illness: A Guide to Understanding Mental Health*

STEVEN L. MASKIN, M.D., *Reversing Dry Eye Syndrome: Practical Ways to Improve Your Comfort, Vision, and Appearance*

MARY JANE MINKIN, M.D., and CAROL V. WRIGHT, Ph.D., *A Woman's Guide to Menopause and Perimenopause*

MARY JANE MINKIN, M.D., and CAROL V. WRIGHT, Ph.D., *A Woman's Guide to Sexual Health*

ARTHUR W. PERRY, M.D., F.A.C.S., *Straight Talk about Cosmetic Surgery*

CATHERINE M. POOLE, with DUPONT GUERRY IV, M.D., *Melanoma: Prevention, Detection, and Treatment*, 2nd ed.

MADHURI REDDY, M.D., M.Sc., and REBECCA COTTRILL, B.Sc.N., *Healing Wounds, Healthy Skin: A Practical Guide for Patients with Chronic Wounds*

E. FULLER TORREY, M.D., *Surviving Prostate Cancer: What You Need to Know to Make Informed Decisions*

BARRY L. ZARET, M.D., and GENELL J. SUBAK-SHARPE, M.S., *Heart Care for Life: Developing the Program That Works Best for You*

Reclaiming Our Health

A Guide to African American Wellness

MICHELLE A. GOURDINE, M.D.

Illustrations by Catharine L. Love

Yale UNIVERSITY PRESS / NEW HAVEN AND LONDON

Published on the foundation established in memory of William Chauncey Williams of the Class of 1822, Yale Medical School, and of William Cook Williams of the Class of 1850, Yale Medical School.

The information and suggestions contained in this book are not intended to replace the services of your physician or caregiver. Because each person and each medical situation is unique, you should consult your own physician to get answers to your personal questions, to evaluate any symptoms you may have, or to receive suggestions for appropriate medications.

The author has attempted to make this book as accurate and up to date as possible, but it may nevertheless contain errors, omissions, or material that is out of date at the time you read it. Neither the author nor the publisher has any legal responsibility or liability for errors, omissions, out-of-date material, or the reader's application of the medical information or advice contained in this book.

Yale University Press books may be purchased in quantity for educational, business, or promotional use. For information, please e-mail sales.press@yale.edu (US office) or sales@yaleup.co.uk (UK office).

Designed by Mary Valencia.
Set in Minion type by Integrated Publishing Solutions, Grand Rapids, Michigan.
Printed in the United States of America by Sheridan Books, Ann Arbor, Michigan.

Library of Congress Cataloging-in-Publication Data
Gourdine, Michelle A., 1962–
      Reclaiming our health : a guide to African American wellness / Michelle A. Gourdine.
            p.   cm. — (Yale University Press health & wellness)
      Includes bibliographical references and index.
      ISBN 978-0-300-14582-3 (clothbound : alk. paper) — ISBN 978-0-300-13705-7 (paperbound : alk. paper) 1. African Americans—Health and hygiene. I. Title.
      RA778.4.A36G385 2011
      362.1089'96073—dc22   2010044397

A catalogue record for this book is available from the British Library.

This paper meets the requirements of ANSI/NISO Z39.48–1992 (Permanence of Paper).

10 9 8 7 6 5 4 3 2 1

*For my mother, Gloria Abram,
my husband, Derek Gourdine, and my children.
This book would not have been possible
without your love, patience, and encouragement.*

CONTENTS

CONTENTS

Every year, tens of thousands of African Americans die from diseases we know how to prevent. This is unacceptable. Frankly, like many of you, I have grown tired of opening the newspaper and reading how African Americans are always the sickest, the latest to be diagnosed, and the earliest to die. For the nearly four hundred years since blacks arrived from the shores of West Africa, we have occupied the lowest rungs on the ladder of health. So how is it that in the decades since the civil rights movement, black men and women have made so much progress politically, educationally, and economically, yet our poor health status persists?

During the fall of 2008, the United States and the world were on the brink of economic disaster. Once-venerable financial institutions were collapsing faster than imploded buildings. Consumers panicked, and the stock market plummeted. "Do something" was the outcry from the public to governmental leaders. In response, the president and his cabinet devised a seven-hundred-billion-dollar plan to "bail out" financial institutions and stabilize our economy. This state of the economy and the plan to repair it were presented to lawmakers in stark and blunt detail. This crisis allowed no time to sugarcoat the facts.

In the same way, I will not gloss over the facts of African American health. We are in full-blown crisis and have been for some time now. The signs of our health crisis were depicted in full relief during my medical training. I treated many black patients who were suffering from complications of chronic disease—mothers relying on dialysis machines to cleanse their bodies from the toxins that their kidneys, damaged by high blood pressure, could no longer handle; wheelchair-bound fathers who lost a leg to diabetes; young women bravely enduring chemotherapy treatments for cancer; grandmothers struggling to climb stairs with painful knees crippled by obesity-related arthritis.

OBSTACLES ON THE PATH TO WELLNESS

It seems illogical that in a country where the life expectancy of all Americans increased by thirty years over the past century, African Americans would remain at such high risk from preventable diseases. So why do we bear a greater burden of disease and death? Some say that lack of health insurance is to blame. Although a higher percentage of African Americans is uninsured compared with whites, almost 80 percent of African Americans have some form of health care coverage. Others suggest that blacks are genetically predisposed to be sicker. Yet race is socially, not genetically assigned. Still others blame African Americans for not taking better care of themselves. But the ability to live a healthy lifestyle is influenced not only by individual motivation but also by environmental resources. Many reasons have been posited, but they all boil down to this: the likelihood of getting a particular disease is ultimately influenced by the number of risk factors you have. African Americans, it turns out, have a higher number of risk factors for virtually every major chronic disease—risk factors such as high obesity rates, low physical activity rates, and so forth. These risk factors are influenced by cultural and social elements that determine what we eat, whether we exercise, how we view ourselves, how we handle stress, and whether we have access to the resources needed to be healthy (that is, income, education, employment, high-quality health care, and safe and supportive neighborhoods).

When I began writing this book in 2006, I was overwhelmed by the volumes of information—hundreds, even thousands of pages of scientific articles, newspaper and magazine articles, chapters of books and entire books, not to mention hundreds of websites—on African American health that have been published. Without question, many authors have attempted to condense this vast body of scientific information into practical advice and recommendations for the African American community. But what makes *Reclaiming Our Health* different is its examination of how African American culture shapes the health choices we make. For many of us, the things we believe, the traditions we treasure, and the values we hold dear influence what we eat, whether we exercise, and when we seek medical attention. For example, cooking big soul food meals is a traditional expression of love. How, then, do we reconcile our need to eat healthier with our desire to enjoy a way of eating that has become an entrenched part of our culture? Must we give up our sense of community and history in order to live healthier lives? Here's another example. African Americans have traditionally celebrated and accepted men and women of all sizes, including those of us who are overweight and obese. How do we reconcile our desire to encourage each other *no matter our size* with the real health threat that extra body weight poses? Must we give up our positive self-image in order to live healthier? This book is my humble attempt to address these important but often ignored obstacles that stand between African Americans and the better health we deserve.

You see, although many of my medical colleagues understand the challenges of African American health on an intellectual level, for me, poor African American health is more than just a concept. I live it every day. I see it at my church on the growing list of members who are sick and shut-in; in my neighborhood, where I see too many little children with big waistlines; in my family, where we have been touched by almost every single leading cause of death. I wrote this book to empower our community to solve our own health problems and save our own lives.

In this book, you will learn easy steps to live a healthier life. Here are just some of the few benefits you'll gain by reading this book and applying its principles to your own life:

- Our traditional diet carries great sentimental meaning, but it places us at higher risk of serious disease. Rather than being scolded about what you shouldn't eat, you will learn how to modify your diet to make it better.
- We all lead hectic and busy lives. This book will show you how to fit the exercise you need into your daily routine.
- Stress has become an all too common part of life. You will learn

healthier ways to cope with stress, including the unique racial stress that African Americans face.

- You will learn how to determine the healthiest weight for you and the best way to reach it.
- By practicing these practical tips, you will leave a legacy of good health and set a positive example for your children and their children.

Reclaiming Our Health starts with a description of our current state of health by answering the following questions:

- Exactly how sick are we?
- Who in our community is at greatest risk of illness?
- Which diseases are primarily responsible for our poor health?

In plain language, Part One establishes our starting point by outlining African Americans' health problems and the main diseases that cause them.

FIVE RISK FACTORS

Part Two moves us toward the goal of reclaiming our health by describing the five leading factors affecting the health of African Americans. Diseases like diabetes and high blood pressure—conditions that are well known in our community—are the end result of obesity, malnutrition, inactivity, toxicity, and social inequity. Four of these factors—obesity, malnutrition, inactivity, and toxicity—address the relationship between our cultural attitudes and beliefs and our health practices. The fifth risk factor, social inequity, addresses the social resources we need to be healthy.

Obesity. As a nation, we're heavier than ever, with two out of every three Americans overweight or obese. But African Americans are the heaviest racial and ethnic group in this country. About eight out of every ten black women and seven out of every ten black men are overweight or obese. If you have too much fat—especially in your waist area—you're at higher risk for heart disease and stroke. Excess weight also raises your blood pressure and blood cholesterol levels, increases your risk for developing diabetes and cancer, and worsens arthritis.

Malnutrition. A healthy diet is necessary to keep the body running smoothly, keep the immune system in top condition, and reduce the risk of chronic diseases. A balanced diet provides the body with the proper combination of vitamins, minerals, and calories. Our traditional soul food diet—full of fat, salt, and calories—contributes to the increased prevalence of disease in the black community. Saturated fat from red meat and fried foods clogs arteries and increases the risk of heart attack or stroke. Salt raises blood pressure, and processed foods high in calories and low in nutrients increase the risk of cancer and contribute to blacks being the heaviest group in the nation.

Inactivity. Regular physical activity lowers blood pressure and cholesterol, prevents diabetes, controls your weight, and relieves depression and anxiety. The recommended level of exercise is thirty minutes of moderate physical activity (for example, brisk walking) per day for most days of the week. But most Americans find it difficult to achieve this level of physical activity, including African Americans. Lack of exercise contributes to obesity, heart disease, diabetes, and high blood pressure.

Toxicity. As a nation, we are overworked and stressed. Working long hours, juggling family responsibilities, and dealing with financial difficulties are major causes of stress. For many African Americans, perceived racism is an added stressor. Chronic stress causes insomnia, elevates blood pressure, raises blood sugar, weakens the body's defenses, and ultimately increases the risk of heart disease, obesity, diabetes, and infections.

Social inequity. The ability to live a healthier life is influenced in part by an environment that supports healthy eating, regular activity, and less stress. African American neighborhoods disproportionately lack these environmental supports.

The chapters of Part Two answer the following questions:

- What is the history behind our food choices?
- What are the main barriers to exercise in our community?

- Does the stress of racism play a role in our health?
- Is our race weaker and genetically predisposed to be sicker?
- How do our living and working environments contribute to our poor health?

Next, each chapter includes a self-assessment to help you determine how the factor is currently affecting your health. Finally, each chapter ends with simple steps you can take to maintain a healthy weight, improve your nutrition, move more, stress less, and improve the health of your community. Reading this section will equip you with the skills to improve your health, and the health of your community.

The final section of this book acknowledges that in addition to self-care, good health also involves getting regular medical care. The chapters in this section show you how to make the most out of your interactions with the health care system by being an informed patient. You will learn how to collect and use your family history to protect your health, how to choose the best doctor for you, and a simple way to understand your options for health care coverage, including an overview of the new health care reform law. Finally, you'll learn the importance of getting regular checkups, even if you believe you are in the best of health.

AN OPPORTUNITY TO REWRITE OUR HEALTH HISTORY

Make no mistake. This book's outline of the reasons for the current state of African American health is not an exercise in finger-pointing or self-pity. No, the purpose of understanding how we got here is to find our way out of our current situation. This book is not a laundry list of things that the government or society must do to help us become healthier; its purpose is not to lay blame, but to empower. As the old saying goes, once you know better, you can do better. The following chapters will provide you with the information you need to make your life better.

What would it look like if all African Americans—men, women, and children—decided to reject our legacy of sickness? If we suddenly decided to create a new legacy of wellness, where would we start? What would we do?

This book offers a clear way to move forward. To be sure, there are many routes to wellness—interstates and side streets, main thorough-fares and unpaved back roads. But for too long, we have been bombarded with unnecessarily complicated blueprints for better health. Here you will find a road map that is simple but not simplistic.

STARTING A LEGACY OF WELLNESS

During our early years in America, our ancestors were excluded from the mainstream health care system and had to rely on a mélange of healers, community organizations, and lay health workers. An assortment of home remedies and health beliefs emerged, and many of these health practices continue today. Yet if we are ever to achieve wellness, we need to renew the way we regard and manage our health.

How do we reverse a trend of unequal health almost four hundred years in the making? One person at a time. Step one is to stop believing the lie that getting sick is inevitable. Each of us has the power to get well and stay well. Step two is to provide the support and encouragement that our loved ones need to make the same choice. Our health status is not only a personal dilemma—it's a community dilemma. We must have both individual and community resolve, and this book will show you how.

We have the power to determine the destiny of our community. Poor health has been our past, but it does not have to be our future. The gap in health status between African Americans and whites is one of our last civil rights frontiers to be conquered. Let's stem the tide of premature dis-ability and death in our community. Our current health condition does not have to be our conclusion. We have work to do. Join me as we begin to go about the business of saving lives. Let's rewrite our health history and reclaim our health.

PART

I

An Unfinished Civil Rights Battle

CHAPTER ONE

An American Injustice: The State of African American Health

Of all the forms of inequality, injustice in health is the most shocking and the most inhuman.
—Dr. Martin Luther King, Jr., March 25, 1966

When I was a medical student some twenty years ago, I encountered a woman I will never forget on my daily rounds. She was in her late fifties and sat, a bit uncomfortably, robed in her hospital gown as a group of my fellow medical students and I surrounded her hospital bed. After obtaining her permission, the attending physician pulled the bedsheet back to reveal the woman's feet. One foot in particular caught our attention. It was charcoal black and somewhat shriveled. We were a bit startled but didn't let on that we were fazed. (After all, we were future doctors. We *had* to appear unruffled!) As the attending doctor questioned her, we discovered that she was a diabetic. Several weeks earlier, a sore had developed on her foot and had not healed. It became infected, the infection spread, and gangrene set in because of the poor circulation in her foot (this is characteristic of diabetics). When one of us asked the woman why she hadn't sought medical attention sooner, she told us that she was afraid of losing her foot. Ironically and sadly, the very thing she feared came to pass.

This woman was one of 2.8 million African Americans living with diabetes. African Americans are more likely to develop diabetes than white Americans, and they are almost three times more likely to undergo amputation. In fact, African Americans are dying at higher rates from every major disease than any other racial or ethnic group in the United States.

As an African American physician, I am particularly struck by the dramatic differences in health between blacks and whites. It seems that every African American has a close friend or family member with diabetes or high blood pressure, and every black family has a member who's overweight or obese, battled cancer, suffered a stroke, or is living with heart disease.

Tremendous advances in medicine have occurred over the past century. Americans live thirty years longer than we did a hundred years ago because of significant improvements in public health, nutrition, and medical care. As a result, all Americans, including African Americans, now have longer and healthier lives. Despite these improvements, the health of black Americans is still worse than the health of white Americans.

This disparity persists some fifty years after the civil rights movement. Because of the sacrifices of many, African Americans have greater educational opportunities than ever before. According to the US Census Bureau, in 2006, 80 percent of African Americans were high school graduates, 2.3 million were enrolled in college, and 1.3 million held an advanced degree.

There are more African Americans in the middle class than ever before. The number of African Americans living in poverty has declined from 31 percent in 1986 to 25 percent in 2008.

The number of black-owned businesses has grown. In 2007, the Census Bureau counted 1.9 million black-owned firms employing more than 920,000 people and generating nearly $137 billion in business revenues.

The political power of African Americans has strengthened. The Congressional Black Caucus has grown from thirteen members in 1971 to forty-three members in 2010. There are more black mayors than at any other time in our nation's history. What's more, our nation has elected the first African American president of the United States.

In the five decades since the civil rights movement began, all Americans have enjoyed better health and lower death rates from the leading causes of death. African Americans made great gains in life expectancy—between 1970 and 2004, black males' life expectancy increased almost ten years compared with white males' increase of eight years. For black females, the increase was eight years compared with white females' increase of five years.

Yet a gap between African American and white American health persists. Blacks still have higher rates of disease and shorter life spans than whites. There are four things you need to know about African Americans' overall health status:[1]

1. Blacks have higher rates of chronic disease than whites.
   - Nearly five of every ten black adults have heart disease. This includes heart attack, stroke, high blood pressure, and hardening of the arteries. African Americans are almost twice as likely to have a stroke as white Americans.
   - African Americans have the highest rate of high blood pressure of all racial and ethnic groups and tend to develop it younger than others.
   - Blacks are about two times more likely than whites to have diabetes.
   - Black men have more cancers of the lung, prostate, colon, rectum, and stomach than white men.
   - Black women are more likely to have colon cancer than white women.
   - Compared to whites, blacks are more likely to be overweight or obese. Seventy percent of African Americans are overweight or obese.

2. Blacks are more likely than whites to suffer from the complications of chronic disease.
   - African Americans have a higher rate of nonfatal stroke, are four to six times more likely than whites to develop high

blood pressure–related kidney failure, and are twice as likely to develop diabetes-related kidney failure.

- African American diabetics are more likely to have a limb amputated than diabetics of other racial and ethnic groups.
- Young African Americans (aged thirty-five to fifty-four) have higher rates of heart attack than white Americans of the same age.
- Blacks are more likely to suffer from heart failure than whites.

3. Blacks have higher death rates from chronic disease than whites.
   - Differences in mortality begin at birth for African Americans. Black infants are two and a half times more likely to die in their first year of life than white infants.
   - Heart disease death rates are 23 percent higher for African Americans than whites, and stroke death rates are 31 percent higher.
   - African Americans are more than twice as likely to die from diabetes as whites.
   - Overall, African Americans are less likely to survive cancer than the general population.
   - Black women are less likely to be diagnosed with, but more likely to die from, breast cancer than white women.

4. Blacks have a shorter life span than whites.
   - The life expectancy at birth for blacks, seventy-three years, is five years shorter than whites and is equal to the life expectancy of whites thirty years ago!

These statistics hit close to home for me because they affect my friends, my family, and myself. My father died at the age of fifty-nine from cancer. My paternal grandmother died at seventy-eight of cancer, and my maternal grandmother died at seventy-five of stroke. My husband was diagnosed with high blood pressure at the age of forty. Several close friends in their forties have diabetes. I could go on . . . .

WE CANNOT AFFORD TO REMAIN SICK

The impact of these diseases goes much deeper than mere statistics suggest. These diseases are destroying the African American community economically and emotionally. Far beyond the 160,000 African Americans who lose their lives each year to chronic disease, black families are being robbed of their ability to achieve the American dream of a better life. Poor health not only causes job loss but is the leading cause of personal bankruptcy.[2] Too many African American families have struggled to make it into the middle class, only to be knocked back down to "poor" by one significant episode of ill health.

The economic impact of African Americans' top health concerns is staggering. The United States spent $2.2 trillion on health care in 2007 (the year for which the most recent data is available). Obesity costs more than $117 billion a year; heart disease costs more than $250 billion a year; cancer costs almost $190 billion a year; stroke costs more than $65 billion a year; diabetes costs more than $170 billion a year; and high blood pressure costs more than $66 billion a year.[3]

We literally cannot afford to be sick. At a time when the jobless rate is rising and the economy is failing, the cost of staying healthy continues to skyrocket. A significant share of rising health care costs is passed along to each of us in the form of higher health care premiums, copayments, and coinsurance. In other words, rising health care costs strain tight household budgets by forcing families to make unfair choices between health care and heating our homes, and between purchasing prescriptions and putting food on the table.

WHY DO OUR HEALTH PROBLEMS PERSIST?

If African Americans' health disparities persist, the consequences are serious. Maintaining the status quo is costly; its toll is emotional and financial. So why hasn't this problem been adequately addressed? We are quick to declare "war" on drug abuse or cancer. Yet no such declaration has accompanied decades of unequal health between blacks and whites. At the height of their outbreak, severe acute respiratory syndrome (SARS), West Nile Virus, avian (bird) flu, the post-9/11 anthrax attacks, and the H1N1 virus received exhaustive media coverage. Anxious Americans took precautions and demanded government action. But if you combined the death tolls from these health crises, they would not even approach the eighty-three thousand excess deaths suffered by African Americans each year—deaths that would not have occurred if the death rate of African Americans was equal to that of whites.[4]

The medical community has certainly documented the problem in depth. Studies such as the Department of Health and Human Services 1985 report on Black and Minority Health and the 2003 Institute of Medicine publication *Unequal Treatment* have demonstrated the health differences between blacks and whites.[5] Hundreds of hours of plenary sessions, workshops, and roundtables at dozens of prominent medical conferences are devoted to this topic each year. Clearly, the medical and public health communities have spent a great deal of time talking about African American health disparities among ourselves. Yet we have done a poor job sharing that information with the public.

Our health problems persist because most Americans, white and black, are unaware of the existence or the magnitude of these racial differences in people's length and quality of life. Few Americans attend medical conferences or regularly read scientific journals and government reports. Most of us rely on the media to highlight important scientific studies. But the media has paid scant attention to the issue of these health disparities. Between 2000 and 2004, the 1,188 minority health articles published in American newspapers represented just 0.09 percent of all health articles published![6]

DOES AFRICAN AMERICAN HEALTH MATTER?

Some may argue that the issue of African American health does not matter to the general population. This view is shortsighted. Minority health inequities will increasingly affect the health and well-being of all Americans because the United States is becoming increasingly diverse. By the year 2050, one of every two citizens will be a person of color.[7] As the United States becomes "browner," the poor health of African Americans will increasingly affect the overall health of the population. Unless we reverse current trends by improving African American health, our country will become a less healthy nation.

THE TOP FIVE

Chronic diseases contribute greatly to the inequality in health status between African Americans and whites. Five diseases in particular—heart disease, stroke, cancer, diabetes, and high blood pressure—are responsible for the greatest numbers of deaths each year in the black community. These are the same top five causes of death for whites, but these diseases affect African Americans out of proportion to our size in the population. Let's take a closer look at these deadly diseases.

WHAT YOU NEED TO KNOW ABOUT HEART DISEASE (HEART ATTACK AND STROKE)

Your heart, a fist-sized bundle of muscle, is responsible for supplying blood to every corner of your body. Blood flows from your heart through a network of blood vessels known as arteries and veins. Together, the heart and blood vessels make up the cardiovascular system.

The formal name for heart disease is "cardiovascular disease." This term actually refers to several diseases of the heart (*cardio*) and blood vessels (*vascular*) that commonly begin as atherosclerosis (or hardening of the arteries) and end in heart attack or stroke. Heart disease is the leading cause of death for men and women worldwide. No other disease kills more African Americans, who are 40 percent more likely to die from heart disease than whites. Since heart disease typically begins with hardening of the arteries, let me explain this condition further.

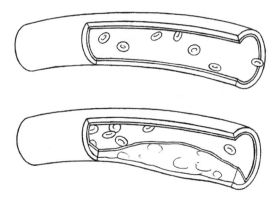

Figure 1. The development of atherosclerosis. A normal artery (top) and an artery blocked by plaque (bottom).

In atherosclerosis, cholesterol and other substances accumulate inside blood vessel walls. This accumulation, known as plaque, is like a pimple under the skin. If the plaque bursts, its contents break through the blood vessel wall, spill into the bloodstream, and trigger the formation of a blood clot at the site of the eruption. Depending on the location of the blood vessel, the clot hampers circulation to the brain, heart, or other organs, depriving them of oxygen and other nutrients. If the blood vessels that supply the heart are blocked by the clot, a heart attack is the result (fig. 1).

Atherosclerosis Causes Heart Attack

In 2009, I moderated a panel discussion featuring three women who survived heart attacks. Although the focus of this panel was on the prevention of heart attacks in black women, the men in the audience also left the meeting with life-saving information.

As each woman shared her remarkable story of survival, three important points recurred:

1. Heart attack is not just a man's disease. According to the National Heart, Lung, and Blood Institute, heart disease kills about half a

million people each year, and women account for nearly half of these deaths. Black women have the highest rates of death from heart disease.

2. Heart attack is not just an old person's disease. Young men and women have heart attacks, too.

3. Surviving a heart attack, for women and men, depends on recognizing its symptoms and trusting your gut. One of the women on my panel went to the emergency room because she felt vaguely uncomfortable. In her words, "I just didn't feel right." The doctor examined her and was ready to send her home, but she refused to leave until she received an EKG. Reluctantly, the doctor complied with her wishes, and to his surprise, the EKG revealed that she was having a heart attack! Her aggressive insistence on being evaluated for heart attack was probably the main difference between her survival and the death of so many people sent home by doctors who fail to accurately diagnose their symptoms.

The most common symptom of heart attack is chest pain, but symptoms can vary widely. Furthermore, women can experience heart attack symptoms that are quite different from those experienced by men (table 1). Recognizing these symptoms is important, because many women have been sent home from the doctor's office with a diagnosis of stress or the stomach flu when they were actually having a heart attack. If you experience any of the symptoms listed in table 1, call 911. Many heart attacks are deadly. Those that aren't lethal can cause severe heart damage, including heart failure.

Atherosclerosis Causes Stroke

A stroke occurs when brain cells die because they are unable to get the blood and oxygen they need. It has two main causes: bleeding into the brain, or blockage of arteries that supply the brain. Atherosclerosis predisposes you to the latter type of stroke. Because blacks are more likely to

Table 1. Symptoms of heart attack

Men	Women
Chest pain radiating to the arms	Heaviness in chest
Sweating	Neck, jaw, shoulder, or back pain
Nausea and vomiting	Nausea and vomiting or abdominal
Lightheadedness or dizziness	pain above the belly button
Upper body pain	Shortness of breath
	Exhaustion or fatigue

have a stroke and die from stroke than whites, every African American should know the warning signs of a stroke:

The National Stroke Association recommends using the F.A.S.T. test to recognize stroke symptoms (table 2).

If you think you're too young to have a stroke, think again. Stroke is not just an older person's disease. In fact, young African Americans are three to five times more likely to suffer a stroke than young whites of the same age. The effects of a stroke can vary from mild to severe to fatal. A stroke can affect a patient's functions in many different ways, depending on the part of the brain affected. For example, stroke patients can have

Table 2. The F.A.S.T. test for stroke

F = Face	Ask the person to smile. Does one side of the face drop?
A = Arms	Ask the person to raise both arms. Does one arm drift downward?
S = Speech	Ask the person to repeat a simple sentence. Does the speech sound slurred or strange?
T = Time	If you observe any of these signs, call 911 or get to the nearest stroke center or hospital.

difficulty with speech, memory, swallowing, balance, coordination, or strength. Many stroke patients lose partial or total function of one side of the body due to weakness or paralysis. Stroke can also cause permanent brain damage.

How to Prevent Heart Disease

Several factors contribute to our increased risk of heart disease. Some of these risk factors are beyond our control, but there is plenty that we can do to control our other risk factors.

Heart disease risk factors we *can't* control:

- Age
- Family history of heart disease

Heart disease risk factors we *can* control:

- Smoking
- High cholesterol
- Type 2 diabetes
- High blood pressure
- Obesity

Type 2 diabetes, high blood pressure, and obesity are interrelated. This means that actions that you take to control one of these conditions have a positive impact on the others. If you decide right now that you are going to add more vegetables to your diet and walk a couple of times a week to take off a few pounds, that decision simultaneously confers the added benefit of keeping your high blood pressure and diabetes under tighter control. Furthermore, making diet and exercise changes to take better care of your body reduces your risk of heart disease.

Cigarette smoking has been shown to speed the progression of atherosclerotic disease by 50 percent. If you don't smoke, you're still at a 20 percent higher risk of progressive atherosclerotic disease if you are regularly exposed to secondhand smoke.[8] Bottom line, both active smoking and exposure to tobacco smoke worsen atherosclerosis, speed its spread throughout your body, and increase your risk of heart attack and stroke. The good news is that when you stop smoking or stop your exposure to secondhand smoke, you decrease your risk of heart disease.

Controlling high cholesterol is a must if you want to reduce your risk of heart disease. Because high cholesterol runs in families, your likelihood of developing atherosclerosis is determined in part by your genetics. But lacking a family history of high cholesterol doesn't earn you a free pass. If you haven't already done so, you need to get a test called a "lipid profile," which checks your total cholesterol, LDL (bad) cholesterol, HDL (good) cholesterol, and triglyceride levels. Normal results are as follows:

Total cholesterol < 200
HDL cholesterol > 60
LDL cholesterol < 100
Triglycerides < 150

LDL, also known as "bad" cholesterol, should be *lower* because this is the type of cholesterol that accumulates inside your blood vessels and increases your likelihood of developing atherosclerosis. Foods that contain saturated fat raise LDL cholesterol levels. This means that every time you eat a steak, cook with butter, or drink whole milk, you are potentially adding an extra layer of cholesterol-laden plaque to the arteries that feed your heart and brain. To combat high LDL levels, replace the saturated animal fat in your diet with healthy fats (table 3).

Your doctor may prescribe medication to lower your LDL cholesterol. Several medications on the market (for example, Lipitor, Zocor, and Crestor) have proven to be effective.

HDL, also known as "good" cholesterol, should be *higher*. It protects you from developing atherosclerosis by preventing LDL from accumulating in your blood vessels. Regular exercise also helps raise HDL cholesterol levels. Red wine (in moderation), green tea, and purple grape juice contain antioxidant chemicals called flavonoids that fight heart disease by raising your level of HDL cholesterol. In addition, cocoa has also been found to be good for your heart. In fact, a 2003 study found that cocoa

Table 3. Replacing bad fats with good fats

Bad fats	Found in . . .	Effect on cholesterol	Increase risk of . . .
Saturated fats	Red meat, butter, whole milk, cheese, bacon	Raise LDL (bad cholesterol)	Heart disease, stroke, high blood pressure
Good fats	Found in . . .	Effect on cholesterol	Decrease risk of . . .
Monounsaturated fats	Nuts, peanut butter, avocado, healthy oils (olive, canola, peanut)	Raise HDL (good cholesterol) and lower LDL (bad cholesterol)	Heart disease, stroke, high blood pressure
Polyunsaturated fats (fish oils, omega-3 fatty acids)	Mackerel, trout, salmon, sardines	Raise HDL (good cholesterol) and lower LDL (bad cholesterol)	Heart disease, stroke, high blood pressure

has higher levels of antioxidants than either red wine or green tea.[9] So why not enjoy grape juice in the morning, green tea in the afternoon, and red wine or hot cocoa (made with cocoa powder, not instant) in the evening for a healthier heart?

Check Your CRP

In addition to controlling your risk factors, consider asking your doctor to check your C-reactive protein (CRP) level. CRP is an indicator of the presence of inflammation in your body. The process of inflammation is believed to cause both the building up of plaque and its bursting through blood vessel walls. It is an important underlying cause of heart disease and can be triggered by many factors, including smoking, overeating, excess fat around the waistline, diabetes, and high blood levels of cholesterol. Elevated CRP levels seem to be a better predictor of future heart attack or stroke than high cholesterol levels.[10] If you have several risk factors for heart disease, ask your doctor to check your high-sensitivity CRP (hs-CRP) level. If your CRP level is high, you can reduce your risk of a future heart attack or stroke by eating a healthy diet, stopping smoking, maintaining a healthy weight, and getting regular exercise. Your doctor may even recommend taking a daily aspirin.

WHAT YOU NEED TO KNOW ABOUT CANCER

Some things in life are so terrible to contemplate that our knee-jerk response is to quickly end the thought with the words, "Heaven forbid!" Like the death of an innocent child or the crash of a plane . . . or the diagnosis of cancer. Being diagnosed with cancer is breathtakingly difficult to fathom. How could a life so full of promise be suddenly threatened by something so dreadful?

Almost twelve years ago, my father's life was forever changed by that terrible diagnosis.

Dad was thin, athletic, and healthy. I don't recall his ever being sick. One day in 1996, my mother called to tell me that my dad had seen the doctor about a cough that wouldn't go away. (I was a practicing doctor in Maryland at the time, and my parents were in Mississippi.) She told me that an X-ray showed fluid on his lungs. I was worried but tried not to let on. I asked my mother what the doctor thought was wrong. She said that test results would return in a few days, but my dad was told that he had either tuberculosis or cancer. I tried to say something encouraging and then hung up the phone and collapsed in my chair. I didn't have to wait for test results. In my heart, I knew that my dad had lung cancer. A few days later, test results proved me right. Eight months later, my father was dead.

Cancer is one of the most terrifying medical diagnoses. Many African Americans of my father's generation are so afraid of this disease that they don't even mention it by name. Instead, they refer to it as "the big C." In fact, I never heard my dad utter the word "cancer." Without a doubt, cancer, the second leading cause of death in this country, is a formidable disease. African Americans with cancer have historically had a higher death rate and shorter survival time of any racial or ethnic group. And as it turns out, my father had one of the most common forms of cancer in African Americans. Other common cancers include colon cancer and prostate cancer. Although breast cancer is less common in African American women, it is more deadly.

Despite these statistics, cancer is *not* an automatic death sentence. With early detection and treatment, more and more people are winning their battles against cancer. High-profile cancer survivors like *Good Morning America* anchor Robin Roberts, poet Nikki Giovanni, Dr. Ben Carson, and former Secretary of State Colin Powell have been able to carry on very active and productive lives after their diagnosis and treatment. Like them, you have the power to conquer this disease by being proactive. As is true in war, the first step in defeating the enemy called "cancer" is to understand what it is and what causes it.

What Is Cancer?

Cells, the building blocks of all living things, go through a normal cycle of growth, division, and death. Cancer occurs when cells develop abnormally and grow uncontrollably. In the same way that uncontrolled weeds can smother the grass in your yard, the uncontrolled growth of cancer cells destroys your normal organs and tissues and interferes with your normal bodily functions. For example, colon cancer can cause tumors (clumps of cells) to grow unrestrained through the walls of the intestines, blocking normal bowel movements, bursting blood vessels, and causing bleeding from the rectum. Cancer metastasizes (spreads) when these abnormal cells enter your bloodstream and are carried to other parts of your body such as the liver, brain, and bones.

What causes your cells to shift from orderly to erratic growth? Although there are many factors, three significant causes are toxic exposures, obesity, and diet. Let me take a moment to explain these.

Toxins and Cancer

Without a doubt, cigarette smoke is the most common and deadly toxic exposure. With each drag of a cigarette, a smoker inhales nearly four thousand chemicals, including carbon monoxide (a deadly gas found in car exhaust and malfunctioning home furnaces), nicotine (the addictive drug found in cigarettes), ammonia (a caustic cleaning fluid), arsenic (found in rat poison), hydrogen cyanide (a deadly substance used in the gas chamber), and formaldehyde (used to preserve dead bodies). No person in his or her right mind would swallow a spoonful of even one of these poisons. Repeated exposure to tobacco smoke causes cancerous changes to occur in normal cells all over the body and results in cancers of the lung, mouth, throat, bladder, cervix, kidney, pancreas, and stomach. According to the American Cancer Society, smoking is also linked to acute myeloid leukemia, a cancer of the blood. As if you needed it, the increased risk of cancer is yet another reason to stop smoking now. Call the American Cancer Society's Quit Line (1-800-QUIT-NOW) for help.

Sunlight is another dangerous exposure. Although our darker skin confers some protection against the sun's ultraviolet rays, black people do get skin cancer. Reggae legend Bob Marley died of a form of skin cancer (malignant melanoma) that grew under his toenail. In fact, African Americans frequently develop skin cancers under our nails and in the webs between our fingers and toes. So, during your annual physical exam, ask your doctor to check your skin closely for evidence of cancerous changes. Furthermore, wear sunscreen daily to protect yourself from sun exposure. Experts recommend that African Americans use sunscreen with an SPF of at least 15 or 30. An added bonus is that sunscreen also makes our skin less likely to develop dark spots (also known as hyperpigmentation) and wrinkles.

Obesity and Cancer

Obesity feeds cancer cells. Excess body fat produces estrogen and other hormones that can accelerate the growth and spread of hormone-sensitive cancers like breast cancer. This is especially significant for African Americans, since more black women die from breast cancer. What's more, elevated insulin levels associated with obesity block an important protein that removes estrogen from circulation. So not only does body fat pump out more estrogen, it also slows the removal of the hormone from the bloodstream. Both of these actions increase the amount of estrogen available to stimulate the growth of breast cancer cells.[11]

Your Diet and Cancer

Does saccharin cause cancer? What about red food dye? If you're confused about what's bad for you and what's not, you have good reason. There has been a lack of consensus on evidence linking these and other substances to cancer. For example, a 2010 report by the Center for Science in the Public Interest says that food dyes increase the risk of cancer, but the Food and Drug Administration has yet to weigh in on the study. Regarding saccharin, although studies conducted in the 1970s showed a link with bladder tumors in laboratory mice, the link to human cancer has not been confirmed. There seems to be clearer evidence that eating certain foods *in excess* increases the risk of cancer. According to the National Cancer Institute, a diet high in processed meats (like hot dogs, bacon, sausage, and cold cuts) increases the risk of death from cancer by about 11 percent. Cancers of the stomach, breast, colon, and prostate have each been linked with the consumption of processed meat. Apparently, the sodium nitrite used to preserve these meats is converted to cancer-causing compounds known as nitrosamines. In addition, regularly eating red meat increases the risk of death from cancer of any type by 20 percent. Specifically, women who eat one and a half servings of red meat or more each day increase their risk of breast cancer twofold. (A serving of red meat is three ounces, or the size of a deck of cards.)[12] You may eat more processed and red meats than you realize. How many times a week do you eat the following?

Breakfast: bacon, sausage, or scrapple

Lunch: pepperoni or sausage pizza, hot dog, burger, or American or Italian cold cut sandwich

Dinner: steak, pork chop, spaghetti with ground beef, or beef stew

It's wise to choose these foods occasionally rather than making them a regular part of your daily meals. Fortunately, there is much more consensus on the types of foods that decrease your risk of cancer; fish and plant-based foods like fresh fruits, vegetables, and whole grains. These foods should form the foundation of your daily meals to reduce your risk of cancer and improve your overall health.

Recognizing Cancer

Another step toward empowering yourself to defeat cancer is to recognize its signs and symptoms. The earlier cancer can be identified, the more treatable it is. Cancer can have any number of signs and symptoms depending on its location.

Breast cancer
- A lump in the breast
- Discharge from the nipple
- Changes in breast shape, size, or skin

Prostate cancer
- Difficulty with urination
- Weight loss
- Pain in lower pelvic area

Colon cancer
- Change in bowel habits
- Blood in stool
- Abdominal pain

With colon cancer, symptoms do not always occur. The best way to detect colon cancer is through regular screening. Talk to your doctor.

Lung cancer

Unfortunately for my father, lung cancer is one of the most difficult cancers to detect early, because it usually has no early symptoms. But early detection is not impossible, especially if you know the common symptoms, which may include:

- Cough
- Chest pain
- Shortness of breath
- Weight loss

Early Detection

Regular cancer screenings are important to prevent cancer or to diagnose it in an early and more treatable stage. The American Cancer Society's current recommendations for prostate, lung, and colon cancer screenings are outlined in table 4.

Although no early lung cancer screening is currently recommended, guidelines may change based on the results of the National Lung Screening Trial, conducted by the National Cancer Institute. This study, in which current and former heavy smokers aged fifty-five to seventy-four were randomly assigned to receive either annual screening CT scans or chest X-rays, was halted in the fall of 2010 because of promising preliminary findings. Study participants who received CT scans had 20 percent fewer lung cancer deaths. As various groups review the study's findings, changes in screening recommendations may be forthcoming. Meanwhile, if you are a current or former heavy smoker, discuss these findings with your doctor.

In 2009, the US Preventive Services Task Force made controversial changes to the recommendations for breast cancer screening (table 5; note: these guidelines do not apply to women at high risk for breast cancer). According to the task force, these changes were meant to strike a balance between the benefits of early detection and the risks of unneces-

Table 4. Screening for colon, prostate, and lung cancer

Colon cancer	Prostate cancer	Lung cancer
Colonoscopy every ten years starting at age 50. African Americans at high risk should start screening at age 40, or	Discuss with your doctor the need for a PSA blood test every year starting at age 45 (or age 40 if strong family history of prostate cancer).	No early screening available.
Flexible sigmoidoscopy every three years, or	Your doctor may also perform a digital rectal exam.	
Barium enema every five years, or		
CT colonography every five years, or		
Your doctor may also perform a fecal occult blood test every year (to look for hidden blood in your bowel movements).		

sary exposure to radiation, additional medical procedures associated with false positive mammograms, and the anxiety and financial costs associated with these risks.

For most women and many health care providers (including me), these "revised" recommendations seemed to contradict the decades spent encouraging women to examine their breasts and get regular mammograms. The new recommendations no longer advise premenopausal women (under the age of fifty) to receive routine mammograms. They also decrease the frequency of mammograms to once every two years for women between the ages of fifty and seventy-four. Furthermore, they discourage breast self-exams and clinical breast exams. My concern is that

Table 5. Screening for breast cancer

Old breast cancer screening guidelines	New breast cancer screening guidelines
Annual mammograms starting at age 40.	No routine mammograms between the ages of 40 and 49. Women between the ages of 50 and 74 should receive mammograms every two years. No mammograms for women 75 years of age and older.
Clinical breast exams at each doctor's visit.	There is no additional benefit to be gained from the clinical breast exam, digital mammogram, or MRI over the regular mammogram.
Women should be taught to perform monthly breast self-exams.	Women should not be taught to perform monthly breast self-exams.

these recommendations, while well-meaning, may place black women at higher risk of dying from breast cancer (as if our death rates weren't high enough). African American women have been historically reluctant to undergo breast cancer screening, but in recent years we have seen an increase in the numbers of African American women getting screened. Furthermore, discouraging routine mammograms in premenopausal black women is worrisome. Black women under the age of forty are more likely than young white women to be diagnosed with breast cancer.[13] These new recommendations are likely to reverse the significant progress we've made toward improving our screening rates and cause our young women to fall between the cracks. So here's my advice: talk to your doctor regarding the type of breast cancer screening you should receive and frequency with which you should receive it. If you will be more at peace

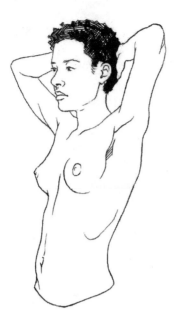

Figure 2. How to self-examine your breasts.
(a) Examine breasts after your menstrual period. Standing in front of a mirror, raise both arms and look at your breasts for dimpling, puckering, discoloration, or other changes in appearance or shape.

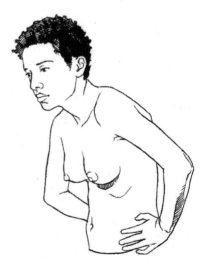

(b) Press hands on hips and look for the same changes.

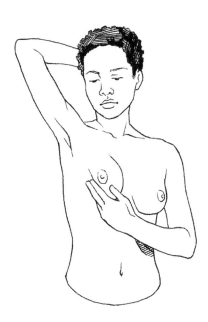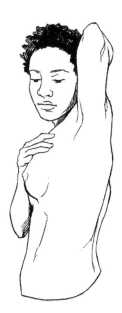

(c) In the shower, raise your right arm over your head and examine entire right breast with your left hand, feeling for unusual lumps, bumps, or tenderness. Also examine under your right arm and collarbone and between your breasts.

(d) Raise your left arm and repeat with your left breast.

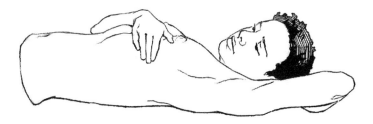

(e) Lie flat with a small pillow under your shoulder. Place your right arm under your head and examine your entire breast for lumps or other abnormalities. Repeat with your left breast.

starting routine mammograms before you turn fifty, let your doctor know. I am forty-seven, and I plan to continue getting regular mammograms. In addition, I see no harm in women continuing to perform a monthly breast self-examination (fig. 2). It allows us to notify our doctors when we detect an abnormality. In many cases, the abnormality won't be cancer, but there are scores of documented cases of women detecting their breast cancer early and increasing their chances for survival.

If you are diagnosed with cancer, several treatment options exist, including surgery, radiation, and chemotherapy. Bottom line, don't let fear stop you from saving your life. Eat a healthy diet, maintain a healthy weight, use sunscreen, stop smoking, get screened, and see your doctor regularly. And remember, the earlier cancer is detected, the greater the chance for a cure.

WHAT YOU NEED TO KNOW ABOUT DIABETES

Diabetes is commonly known as "the sugar" in the African American community, but there's nothing sweet about it. It is the seventh leading cause of death in the United States. People with diabetes, including four of every ten African Americans, have double the risk of death (primarily from heart disease) compared to people of similar age without the disease.

Diabetes is a condition in which the blood sugar is too high. In normal circumstances, your body converts the food you eat into sugar, which the cells use as a source of fuel. A hormone called insulin acts as a key that unlocks your cells and allows sugar to enter them from your bloodstream. In diabetes, the body either does not produce enough insulin or does not respond to insulin. In either instance, sugar builds up in the blood, too little sugar enters the cells, and ultimately the body doesn't get the fuel it needs. Sugar in the blood is like sunburn to the skin—it causes premature aging of blood vessels and makes them ripe for the development of atherosclerosis (hardening of the arteries) and heart disease. Heart attacks are much more common in people with diabetes than in the general population. But the blood vessel damage caused by diabetes does not stop with the heart. It also damages the blood vessels of the eyes, kidneys, and limbs. That's why people with diabetes develop blindness, experience kidney failure, and lose limbs to amputation.

The three types of diabetes are type 1, type 2, and gestational diabetes.

Type 1 diabetes

In type 1 diabetes, the pancreas produces little to no insulin. People with type 1 diabetes are born with the condition, which is usually diagnosed in childhood. About 5 to 10 percent of people with diabetes have type 1 diabetes.

Gestational diabetes

Gestational diabetes occurs in women during pregnancy and usually disappears after the birth of the baby. Women with gestational diabetes have an increased risk of developing type 2 diabetes within five to ten years.

Type 2 diabetes

Unlike type 1 diabetes, which is caused by an inherited inability to produce insulin, type 2 diabetes is directly related to obesity and accounts for 95 percent of the estimated 3.7 million cases of diabetes among African Americans.[14] Here are the signs and symptoms of diabetes:

- Feeling tired or ill
- Blurred vision
- Frequent infections
- Slow-healing wounds
- Excessive thirst
- Excessive urination
- Weight loss
- *No symptoms at all:* about a third of African Americans with diabetes don't know they have it

You are at greater risk of type 2 diabetes if you are overweight, especially around the waist. If you are a female whose waist measures more than thirty-five inches in diameter, or a male whose waist measures more than forty inches, your urine should be checked for excess sugar every three years. Prediabetes also increases the risk for type 2 diabetes. In this condition, blood sugar levels are higher than normal (that is, a fasting blood sugar between 100 and 125) but not yet high enough for a diagnosis of diabetes. With regular exercise and a healthy diet, progression to diabetes can be prevented.

Diabetes may seem harmless. After all, many people with diabetes have no symptoms of the disease for years. But diabetes is a serious disease. If blood sugar levels are not stabilized, the consequences are disabling and life-threatening. By far the biggest danger is heart disease, the cause of death for eight of every ten people with diabetes. In addition, three of every four diabetics have high blood pressure. African American diabetics are more likely than white diabetics to suffer serious complications from the disease:

- Blacks are almost 50 percent more likely to go blind (a condition called diabetic retinopathy)
- Blacks are three to five times more likely to suffer from kidney disease, often resulting in dialysis and transplant
- Blacks are almost three times more likely to suffer from lower-limb amputations

Know Your Numbers

If you have type 2 diabetes, you and your doctor can keep your condition under control by knowing three numbers:

1. Your blood sugar,
2. Your waist measurement, and
3. Your blood pressure.

Eating a proper diet, getting regular exercise, and maintaining a healthy weight will help you keep these numbers in check, sometimes without needing medication.

WHAT YOU NEED TO KNOW ABOUT
HIGH BLOOD PRESSURE

If you don't feel sick, does that mean you're healthy? Not necessarily. For millions of African Americans with high blood pressure, dangerous changes are taking place in their bodies, but they're not aware of them. That's why high blood pressure is known as the "silent killer."

High blood pressure is like a dishonest mechanic who sneakily disconnects a hose here and loosens a screw there so that the vehicle that is your body looks and runs just fine for the short term. But one day when you least expect it, all systems come to a screeching halt. In the case of high blood pressure, those systems are your heart, your brain, and your kidneys.

Two out of every five African Americans have high blood pressure—more than any other racial or ethnic group in the world. Imagine attending a family reunion with fifty of your closest relatives . . . twenty of them have high blood pressure, and many of them have no idea that they do.

What Is High Blood Pressure?

High blood pressure, or hypertension, results when the force of blood against the walls of your blood vessels is too strong. It causes your heart to work harder than it should to pump blood throughout your body.

Blood pressure is stated in two numbers. For example, my blood pressure is around 110/70 (say "110 over 70"). The top number, 110, is my systolic blood pressure. This number represents the force of my blood against blood vessel walls when my heart beats. The bottom number, 70, is my diastolic blood pressure. This number represents the force of my blood against blood vessel walls when my heart relaxes between beats.

Normal blood pressure is lower than 120/80. High blood pressure is 140/90 or higher. If your blood pressure is between 120/80 and 140/90, you have borderline high blood pressure or "prehypertension" (table 6).

Every adult's blood pressure should be measured a minimum of once every two years starting at age twenty-one. If your blood pressure is high, get it checked at every doctor's visit.

Table 6. Blood pressure levels	
Normal blood pressure	Lower than 120/80
Prehypertension (borderline high blood pressure)	120/80 to 139/89
Hypertension (high blood pressure)	140/90 or higher

Risk Factors for High Blood Pressure

The following factors increase your risk for getting high blood pressure:

- African American
- Obesity
- Smoking
- Physical inactivity
- Family history of high blood pressure

Although young people can also get the disease, your risk for high blood pressure increases as you age.

Each of these risk factors is important, but there are three other surprising reasons your blood pressure may be elevated—hidden salt, prescription and over-the-counter medications, and illicit drug use.

Salt

A diet high in salt overloads the body with sodium. In an attempt to wash out the excess sodium, the body retains water, which raises blood pressure. African Americans tend to be more sensitive to the effect of salt on blood pressure. In fact, 73 percent of African Americans with high blood pressure are salt-sensitive, meaning that salt raises our blood pressure higher than in whites. Research suggests that this salt sensitivity can be explained in part by genetics.[15]

The American Heart Association recommends consuming no more than one teaspoon of salt a day (2,300 mg of sodium). But the average

American consumes at least three times as much salt. It's not difficult to eat more salt than you realize, because eliminating extra salt from your diet requires more than simply removing the salt shaker from the dinner table. Salt is a popular preservative found in practically every canned, boxed, processed, or restaurant food.

To avoid hidden salt, prepare your own foods at home from scratch. That way, you have complete control over the amount of salt in your food. If you do order take-out, ask that your foods not be seasoned with monosodium glutamate (MSG), which is high in sodium. Also check the labels of packaged foods for sodium and choose foods that contain less than 5 percent of the percent value (% Daily Value) of sodium per serving.

Medications and Drugs

Several types of medication can raise blood pressure (table 7). These include prescription birth control pills, steroids, antidepressants, and pain relievers. Some over-the-counter pain relievers raise blood pressure because they contain sodium (for example, naproxen sodium or sodium salicylate) or caffeine (for example, Excedrin). Over-the-counter decon-

Table 7. Medications and drugs of abuse that may elevate blood pressure

Prescription medications	Over-the-counter medications	Drugs of abuse
Birth control pills	Headache medicines containing sodium	Powder cocaine
Steroids	Headache medicines containing caffeine	Crack cocaine
Antidepressants	Diet pills	Alcohol
Pain medications	Cold or allergy medicines containing pseudoephedrine	
	Cold or allergy medicines containing phenylephrine	

gestants, cold and allergy medications, and some diet pills contain pseudoephedrine and phenylephrine, ingredients that raise blood pressure by causing the heart to beat faster. Check labels carefully.

Certain drugs of abuse—specifically cocaine and crack—and excessive alcohol use also raise blood pressure.

Why Diagnose and Treat High Blood Pressure?

Although high blood pressure may produce no symptoms, it is dangerous for two main reasons:

1. It increases the risk for heart failure by making the heart work too hard, and
2. The high force of blood flow damages blood vessels and organs, setting the stage for heart disease, stroke, and kidney failure (including dialysis or transplant).

Heart attack and stroke are the most common and most deadly outcomes of high blood pressure, and African Americans have a higher risk of all high blood pressure–related complications.

How to Treat High Blood Pressure

High blood pressure is a disease that responds well to changes in lifestyle. It is essential to follow a sensible diet and exercise regimen if you've been diagnosed. If you're overweight, losing weight can help keep blood pressure under control. Finally, if you have been prescribed blood pressure medication, you *must* take it every day, whether you feel sick or not. Skipping your medication is like playing Russian roulette with your health.

CONQUERING OUR HEALTH CHALLENGES

Now that you have a better understanding of the diseases that most commonly affect African Americans, it's time to learn more about the common factors that cause them. Five common risk factors are to blame. Controlling these factors is not hard; learning how to control them is the focus of Parts Two and Three of this book.

II

Rewriting Our Health History
A New Vision of Better Health

CHAPTER TWO

Lose Weight and Win:
Fighting Obesity

Two-thirds of all Americans are overweight or obese. But if you relied on pop culture as an accurate barometer of American society, you'd never know it. Magazines, movies, and the media say "thin is in!" Skeletal actresses prance down red carpets, revealing ribs and collarbones with every flash of the camera. Stick-thin fashion models live on diet sodas and cigarettes to achieve success in an industry where a size 4 is considered obese.

Yet full-figured black actresses and models like Tyra Banks, Queen Latifah, and Mo'Nique have gained fame and fortune while bucking conventional trends. This apparent contradiction can be explained by fundamental differences in cultural attitudes toward body weight. The black community, showing its individuality by going against the societal grain, accepts, embraces, and—in some instances—favors large body sizes. Some black men prefer women with a little "meat on their bones." And many black women agree that bodies with Rubenesque curves are more attractive.[1] Furthermore, some African Americans still uphold the outdated belief that carrying a little extra weight is advantageous in the event of illness, providing a "reserve"—an extra level of protection against sickness—that being thin doesn't provide.

Despite these affirming attitudes, there's no denying that excess body fat is unhealthy. Obesity places undue stress on your heart and lungs. It wears out your joints, slowly robs you of your mobility and independence, and destroys your body's normal metabolism. And more than any other race or gender, black women are most affected by obesity and conditions directly related to obesity.

Most black women are fully aware that obesity poses serious health risks. Concerns about the negative impact of weight on health, a wish to appear more attractive, and a desire for greater stamina and mobility (that is, the ability to climb stairs without pain or to play with children and grandchildren) are the leading reasons why overweight and obese black women personally prefer to be a more healthy weight.[2] Yet black women who have made the decision to lose weight are often surprised to find a lack of support among their closest family and friends. I have even fallen into this trap. Several months ago, a friend of mine announced that she was going to try to lose a few pounds. Without even thinking, I immediately responded, "Girl, you look fine. You don't need to lose weight." I surprised myself by that comment, because I knew that losing a few pounds would benefit her, not harm her. So why did I say that? My remark grew out of a deeply ingrained, culturally based desire to boost my friend's self-esteem by not making her feel bad about her body size. Black women do this all the time. Our intent is to encourage each other, to show that our love and acceptance of each other is not predicated on how much we weigh.

But sometimes we go too far. When it comes to maintaining a healthy weight, we are often our own worst enemies. Some comments directed toward black women who've changed their exercise and eating habits in an attempt to lose weight can be pretty mean. Instead of hearing their healthier lifestyle praised, some women receive comments like, "You're wasting away!" or "You look sickly!" Well-meaning or not, these comments can discourage women from achieving a healthier weight.

It's no wonder that black women who are trying to balance cultural pressures to embrace their curves with valid concerns about their health are downright double-minded about their weight. Yo-yo dieting and failed attempts at weight loss are the result.

African Americans' complicated and often contradictory cultural beliefs and expectations about body size are major barriers to maintaining a healthy body weight. Once African Americans begin to take the health risks of obesity more seriously, the number of premature deaths in our community will decrease.

You might wonder why my opening remarks focus on the weight of black women when the waistlines of American adults of all races and genders are expanding. My rationale is simple. Although obesity and overweight are at epidemic proportions in this country, no group is affected more severely than African American women. Eight of every ten black women are overweight, and half of all black women are obese. These figures exceed the national average by 14 and 20 percentage points, respectively.

Black men have a weight problem, too. Sixty-seven percent of black men are overweight, and 31 percent are obese. These figures mirror the national averages for overweight and obesity in the United States.

Whether you are female or male, excess body fat is more than just a matter of outward appearance. It is a significant health threat that is associated with heart disease, stroke, high blood pressure, diabetes, and some forms of cancer. Therefore, it should come as no surprise that black men and women are more likely to have type 2 diabetes, high blood pressure, and stroke, and black women have a higher prevalence of heart disease—all obesity-related diseases that kill thousands each year.

WHAT IS OBESITY?

Obesity is simply an excessive amount of body fat, roughly 30 percent over your ideal weight. It is most commonly measured using the body mass index, a tool that considers your weight relative to your height. The body mass index, or BMI, provides a range of weights for height that represent underweight, normal weight, overweight, and obese. Overweight and obesity denote a level of body fat that places your health in danger.

Where you carry your body fat is as important as the amount of body fat you have. A "spare tire" increases your risk of heart disease and diabetes. If you have a waist circumference greater than thirty-five inches (female) or forty inches (male), your risk of disease is higher, and here's why. More than just a harmless extra layer of padding, excess abdominal fat destroys the body's normal functioning by altering our insulin metabolism and hormone production and damaging the cardiovascular system. Read on. You may be shocked to learn just how dangerous fat is.

Fat Causes Insulin Resistance and Diabetes

That type 2 diabetes is associated with obesity is a well-known fact. We are now beginning to understand what's behind that association—a process known as insulin resistance. Here's how it works (fig. 3). During digestion, much of what you eat and drink is broken down into glucose (sugar). When sugar enters the bloodstream, the pancreas secretes a hormone called insulin that removes sugar from the blood by escorting it into cells, where it is converted into energy. Fat cells disrupt that process by releasing chemicals that make cells less responsive to normal amounts of insulin. This lack of responsiveness to normal amounts of insulin is known as insulin resistance. As a result, the pancreas is required to produce higher than normal levels of insulin to remove sugar from the blood.[3] Eventually, the pancreas, exhausted by being chronically overworked in the presence of excess body fat, is no longer able to pump out enough insulin to compensate for insulin resistance. Blood sugar levels rise, and diabetes results.

Fat Causes Atherosclerosis

If that's not enough to convince you that body fat is dangerous, consider this. The elevated levels of insulin and sugar circulating in the blood not only set the stage for diabetes but also damage the delicate lining of blood

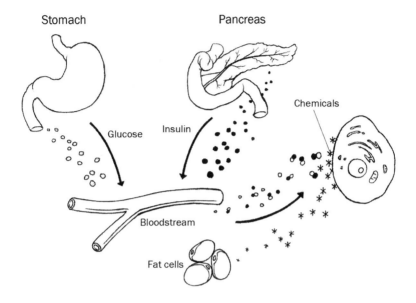

Figure 3. Fat cells cause insulin resistance by releasing chemicals that block entry of glucose and insulin into cells.

vessels. Think of it this way: if you scrape your knee, it is more susceptible to infection because germs can enter through the break in the skin. In like manner, the irritation caused by excess insulin and sugar in the blood creates a break in blood vessel walls that allows cholesterol-laden plaque to enter and accumulate. If that isn't enough, fat tissue also releases chemicals that trigger chronic low-grade inflammation and accelerate the hardening of arteries.[4] Both processes cause high blood pressure, heart disease, and stroke by creating a more favorable environment for the buildup of plaque in blood vessels that can eventually block blood flow to the heart and brain.

Fat Is Associated with Metabolic Syndrome

If you carry excess weight around your abdomen (as measured by your waist circumference), there is a strong possibility that you may have metabolic syndrome. This is a cluster of signs that in combination significantly increase your risk of type 2 diabetes, heart attack, and stroke. The most common trio of signs is abdominal obesity, high blood pressure, and elevated blood sugar. According to the American Heart Association, if you have three or more of the following signs, you have metabolic syndrome:

- A blood pressure equal to or greater than 130/85 mm Hg
- A fasting blood sugar equal to or greater than 100 mg/dl
- A waist circumference equal to or greater than forty inches (male) or thirty-five inches (female)
- A low level of HDL (good) cholesterol, less than 40 if you are male or less than 50 if you are female
- A triglyceride (blood fat) level equal to or greater than 150 mg/dl

If your waist circumference exceeds the limits listed above, ask your doctor to check your blood pressure, blood sugar, and lipid profile (which measures cholesterol and triglycerides) to determine whether you have metabolic syndrome. If you meet the criteria, there are four things you can do right now to decrease your risk of serious illness:

1. Lose weight. A loss of 7 to 10 percent of your body weight (approximately ten pounds) will reduce your disease risk.
2. Walk thirty minutes a day for five to seven days out of every week.
3. Eat a healthy diet of predominantly fish, fruits, vegetables, and whole grains to lower your cholesterol and blood pressure. Take medicines as prescribed.
4. If you smoke, stop.

Other Health Consequences of Obesity

It's ironic that one of the terms black folks use for overweight is "healthy," because there's nothing healthy about it. If you are overweight or obese, chances are that you don't feel good. Carrying around excess weight can leave you short of breath and out of energy. The pressure that extra weight places on your joints is crippling; arthritis leaves you unable to play with your children or even get up and down the stairs of your home without pain. Every extra pound you gain places up to three pounds of stress on your knees and hips when you walk, and up to ten pound of stress on those joints when you run. Many people who are overweight have a large amount of fatty tissue in their throat that can block their windpipe. This condition, known as sleep apnea, can stop your breathing several times a night and cause drowsiness during the day. It also increases your risk of heart disease and stroke.

Even if you feel fine now, the long-term effects of excess weight on your health are harmful. High blood pressure is twice as common in obese adults, and more than 80 percent of diabetics are overweight or obese. Obesity also raises the levels of cholesterol in your blood, increasing your risk of heart disease.

You don't have to gain a large amount of weight to affect your health negatively. People who gain only eleven to eighteen pounds over their desired weight increase their risk of developing type 2 diabetes to twice that of those who have not gained weight. In addition, for every two pounds you gain, you increase your risk of developing arthritis by 9 to 13 percent.

WHAT CAUSES OBESITY?

Three important factors contribute to our obesity epidemic:

1. Overeating. You gain weight when you store more calories as fat than you burn. So obviously, the quality of your diet and your level of physical activity play a role.
2. Genetics. Your heredity determines how your body burns calories and stores fat. That's why some people seem to be able to eat almost anything and never gain weight while the rest of us gain weight much more easily.
3. Culture. Our African American culture has a more full-figured perception of what is thought to be attractive.

Overeating

Your weight is the result of the balance between the calories you consume and store as fat (that is, what you eat) and the calories you burn (that is, how much you move). A calorie is simply a unit of energy that is provided by the nutrients—carbohydrates, fats, and protein—that you eat and drink. Bread and pasta are composed primarily of carbohydrates, which when broken down provide 4 calories per gram. Nuts, beans, and lean meat are good sources of protein, which when broken down also provide 4 calories per gram. Mayonnaise, butter, and cooking oil are composed mostly of fat, which when broken down provides 9 calories per gram.

Calories are to the body as gasoline is to a car—both provide fuel. But unlike a gas tank, which has a finite capacity for gas, the body will take in as many calories as you feed it and store the excess as fat. That's why it's important to eat only as many calories as your body needs. The actual number of calories your body needs depends on your level of activity and takes into account three factors:

1. Basal metabolic rate. This represents the amount of energy your body needs to perform automatic functions at rest, such as breathing, pumping blood, and blinking eyelids. You may be surprised to know that these functions account for about 60 percent of the total calories burned each day.
2. Physical activity. Walking, raking, sweeping, and lifting are some of the physical activities that most of us perform every day. The amount of additional energy your body needs to perform these functions represents about 30 percent of the total calories burned each day. The more intense the activity, the more calories needed.
3. Digestion. Energy is needed to break down the food that you eat. Digestion accounts for about 10 percent of the total calories burned each day.

Your basal metabolic rate, physical activity level, and digestion determine the number of calories you burn each day. If you burn more calories than you eat, you lose weight. If you burn fewer calories than you eat, the excess energy is stored as body fat and you gain weight.

How Many Calories Do You Need?

The average adult needs approximately 2,000 calories per day with the following caveats:

1. Men need more calories than women.
2. Younger people need more calories than older people.
3. More active people need more calories than less active people.
4. Heavier people need more calories than thinner people. (Yes, you read that right!)

Genetics

If you are overweight or obese, you are probably not the only one in your family struggling with weight. Whether you are big-boned or petite, I bet you can identify other family members with the same build.

Coincidence?

Hardly.

Genetic factors (or heredity) influence how your body stores fat and burns calories. Through heredity, your parents pass down traits that govern everything about you, including the rate at which you burn calories (your metabolism). If your metabolism is fast, you burn calories quickly. If it is slow, you burn calories slowly. Therefore, it is not surprising that obesity tends to run in families. Regardless of your current weight, if you have overweight or obese family members, your shared family history predicts that your metabolism may be slower. This means that you may be more likely to be overweight, but it does not guarantee that you will be overweight if you use your knowledge of your family history to your advantage by counting calories more closely and exercising more diligently.

Cultural Attitudes and Perceptions

By now you should have a good understanding of what obesity is, what causes it, and why it's dangerous. For some, this information may be sufficient motivation to attain or maintain a healthy weight. Yet more than BMI, genetics, and metabolism, a healthy weight requires the right mind-set. Cultural attitudes and beliefs frame the way we perceive ourselves and therefore affect our motivation to lose weight . . . or not. Let me explain.

African Americans and Caucasians view "healthy weight" very differently. In general, the ideal body type is thinner for whites than for blacks. The African American community does not tend to buy into the near-anorexic ideal portrayed by pop culture. A classic study reviewing data from the 1985 National Health Interview Survey further illustrates the importance of viewpoint. This study showed that overweight black women are less likely than overweight white women to perceive that their weight is unhealthy. This sounds strange until you realize that many black women tend to compare their weight to other black women. If most of your peers are heavier than average, it stands to reason that you would consider your weight to be "normal" by comparison.[5] An overweight woman who perceives her weight to be normal is less likely to be motivated to lose weight; she simply does not see the need.

IS BMI VALID FOR AFRICAN AMERICANS?

Although the standard measure for healthy weight is the BMI, this tool is not without its skeptics. My speeches have allowed me to interact with audiences across the country, and I have found that many African Americans believe that the body mass index (BMI) measurement is not applicable to our race. During more than one question-and-answer session, black audience members have asked me whether the BMI is valid for the African American "body type." The implication is that the African American "build" is meant to carry more weight. I believe that this question stems from a widely held view in our community that African Americans are naturally larger. This is not true. The truth is that there is no one body type that is specifically African American; black men and women can be found in a wide range of body frames from small to large. And in general, standard definitions for overweight and obesity are valid regardless of your body frame. The perception that blacks are "naturally" larger perpetuates overweight and obesity.

CHANGING OUR MINDSET

To achieve real and lasting positive changes in our health, African Americans must relinquish our ranking atop the obesity charts by aligning our beliefs about weight with the facts. Losing weight can help prevent all of our leading causes of disease and death. Weight loss can lower blood sugar in

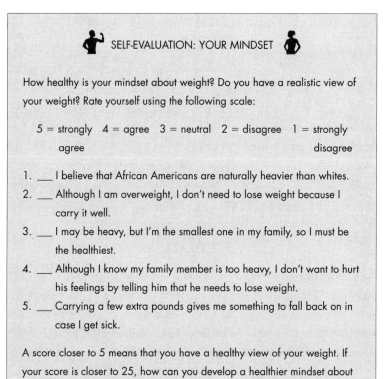

SELF-EVALUATION: YOUR MINDSET

How healthy is your mindset about weight? Do you have a realistic view of your weight? Rate yourself using the following scale:

5 = strongly   4 = agree   3 = neutral   2 = disagree   1 = strongly
    agree   disagree

1. ___ I believe that African Americans are naturally heavier than whites.
2. ___ Although I am overweight, I don't need to lose weight because I carry it well.
3. ___ I may be heavy, but I'm the smallest one in my family, so I must be the healthiest.
4. ___ Although I know my family member is too heavy, I don't want to hurt his feelings by telling him that he needs to lose weight.
5. ___ Carrying a few extra pounds gives me something to fall back on in case I get sick.

A score closer to 5 means that you have a healthy view of your weight. If your score is closer to 25, how can you develop a healthier mindset about your weight and body image? Keep reading and discover how our community can begin to change our mindset about overweight and obesity.

people with diabetes, control blood pressure in people with high blood pressure, and lower LDL (bad) cholesterol and raise HDL (good) cholesterol.

WE MUST ACKNOWLEDGE THE TRUTH

Excess body weight is more than a matter of vanity or preference. It is responsible for all five of the top killers of African Americans and has devastated our community. The majority of black men and women are overweight or obese, and the consequences are deadly. Everyone who cares about improving our health and the health of generations to come must understand that carrying excess weight is like walking around with a ticking time bomb. Our community can no longer afford to embrace unhealthy body weights.

Although you may be accepting of your current weight, it may not be healthy. For some, there is no question that your weight is unhealthy because you have already been diagnosed with high blood pressure, diabetes, or other obesity-related health problems. But what if you feel fine despite a few extra pounds? Even though you may feel and look like the picture of health, your weight may be setting you up for future health problems. That's why it's so important to ensure that your weight reaches and stays in the healthy range.

WHAT'S YOUR HEALTHY WEIGHT?

According to the National Heart Lung and Blood Institute, your BMI, waist-hip ratio, and risk factors for obesity-related diseases help determine whether your weight is healthy. Right now, get out your tape measure and your scale, and follow the three steps outlined below to determine whether your weight falls in the healthy range.

- Calculate your BMI
- Calculate your waist-hip ratio
- Determine your family risk

Table 8. Calculating your BMI

$$BMI = \frac{\text{weight in pounds} \times 703}{\text{height in inches}^2}$$

So if your weight is 155 pounds and you are 5'5" (or 65"),
your BMI would be:

$$\frac{155 \times 703}{65 \times 65}$$

$$= 25.8 \text{ (overweight)}$$

Calculate Your Body Mass Index

As you learned earlier in this chapter, the body mass index (BMI) measurement uses your height and weight to estimate how much body fat you have, and classifies your weight as normal, overweight, or obese (tables 8, 9).

Calculate Your Waist-Hip Ratio

Excess weight around your waist places you at higher risk for heart disease and diabetes. So having a goal of obtaining six-pack abs—or at least a two-pack—is not just vanity. In fact, carrying excess fat around your

Table 9. BMI levels

BMI	Considered to be . . .
Less than 18.5	Underweight
18.5 to 24.9	Normal
25 to 29.9	Overweight
30 or higher	Obese

midsection is more dangerous than carrying excess weight on your hips and thighs. Simply put, a potbelly is more hazardous to your health than cellulite! Furthermore, excess belly fat increases your risk of disease even if your BMI falls in the "normal" range.

Earlier in this chapter, you learned that a waist circumference of more than thirty-five inches in women or forty inches in men increases your risk of disease. A more precise measurement is the waist-hip ratio. It requires only a tape measure and can be calculated in three easy steps:

1. Wrap the tape measure around your waist at the belly button and write down the number in inches.
2. Wrap the tape measure around the widest part of your hips (below your pelvis) and write down the number in inches.
3. Divide the waist measurement by the hip measurement to get your waist-hip ratio.

A healthy waist-hip ratio is 0.8 or less in women, and 0.9 or less in men. So if you are a man whose waist measurement is thirty-two inches and your hip measurement is thirty-six inches, your waist-hip ratio is 0.89 (healthy range). A risky waist-hip ratio is 1.0 or more in women or men. If your waist-hip ratio is 1.0 or more, you can lower your ratio simply by eating right and getting more exercise.

WHAT'S YOUR FAMILY RISK?

Heredity plays an important role in predicting your body size. This doesn't mean that your obese relatives have doomed you to being obese, but it does mean that your risk of being obese or developing obesity-related diseases is greater.

To assess your family risk, answer the questions below. Every "yes" increases your risk for obesity-related diseases like high blood pressure, heart attack, stroke, and diabetes. If you or members of your family have any of these conditions, you should work even harder to maintain a healthy weight.

1. Do you or does a member of your family have high blood pressure?
2. Have you or has a family member had a heart attack?
3. Have you or has a family member had a stroke?
4. Do you or does a member of your family have diabetes or high blood sugar?
5. Do you or does a member of your family have high LDL (bad) cholesterol?
6. Do you smoke?
7. Do you exercise less than thirty minutes a day most days of the week?

If you discover that you are at high risk, here's what you need to do next.

Lose ten pounds.

Yes, ten pounds. If you think that ten is a convenient number that I pulled out of the air, you're wrong. Studies have shown that losing just 5 to 7 percent of your body weight (roughly ten pounds for people weighing two hundred pounds or less) can dramatically improve your health. If you have already been diagnosed with type 2 diabetes, losing ten pounds can lower your blood sugar and help you get off medication. If you have high blood pressure, losing ten pounds helps you keep it under control; it also lowers LDL (bad) cholesterol and raises HDL (good) cholesterol.

HOW NOT TO LOSE TEN POUNDS

There is no shortage of weight-loss options. Many best-selling books describe every type of diet imaginable, and television infomercials sell all kinds of weight-loss pills, exercise equipment, and fitness videos. These get-skinny-quick schemes can be very tempting. Who doesn't like immediate gratification? So, before I tell you what works, you first need to know what's not worth your time.

Fad Diets

Diet books are some of the most popular books on the market today. It seems that people are hungry for the quick weight loss these books claim to offer. The promises of some of these diets make absolutely no sense. They claim that you can "Eat all you want and lose weight!" That's impossible. If you eat more calories than you burn, you will gain weight.

Other plans eliminate certain foods or entire food groups or overemphasize a particular food as the key to losing weight. For example, one extremely popular diet eliminates carbohydrates. Another one centers on eating several servings of grapefruit or grapefruit juice each day. It is possible to lose weight quickly on these types of diets, but you will be left with several serious problems:

1. Nutritional deficiency. The cornerstone of a well-balanced diet is eating a variety of foods. These diets lack variety. Because they often focus on certain foods, they are deficient in important vitamins, minerals, and nutrients. These nutritional deficiencies can weaken your immune system, leaving you vulnerable to disease.
2. Muscle loss. If you achieve the quick weight loss that these diets promise, you have likely lost water weight and precious muscle (especially if you don't exercise).
3. Weight regain. Many of these diets are boring because of their lack of variety. They are difficult to sustain over the long run, which makes it more likely that you will regain the weight you lost.

It is better to lose weight by adopting healthy eating habits than to pursue crash diets (table 10). So, how can you tell whether a particular diet plan makes sense for you?

1. The diet should not eliminate an entire category of food or nutrient. The diet should allow you to eat from all foods groups.
2. The diet should not require that you skip meals.

Table 10. Comparison of diet plans

Fad diet	Healthy diet
Focuses on one food or food group (e.g., cabbage, no carbs), resulting in nutritional deficiencies	Encourages a variety of foods to ensure proper nutrient balance
Encourages fasting, starvation, and skipping meals, which slows down the rate at which you burn fat	Three meals and two to three healthy snacks per day are recommended to keep your metabolism high
Promises dramatic weight loss (lose forty pounds in a month!); more likely to regain weight	Gradual weight loss (one to two pounds per week); more likely to keep weight off

3. Weight loss should be gradual—that is, one to two pounds per week.
4. Most important, the diet should be something you can honestly maintain over the long term. You should be able to make that way of eating a way of life for you.

"Fat-Burning" and Diet Pills

Lose weight in your sleep! Eat as much as you want and lose weight! These are just some of the breathless claims from the makers of these weight-loss pills. They sound too good to be true . . . and they usually are! Most "fat-burning" pills are classified as dietary supplements; therefore approval by the Food and Drug Administration (FDA) is not required. Without FDA oversight, there are no quality controls on the content of these supplements, so you don't really know what you're taking.

Some of these supplements contain herbs that have a diuretic effect, which means that they help you lose water weight, but they do not burn fat. Many so-called fat-burning pills contain ephedra or ma-huang, ingredients that increase your heart rate and can be especially dangerous if you have a heart condition or high blood pressure.

All in all, these get-thin-quick pills appeal to the desire to lose pounds quickly and easily. They may help you lose a few pounds, but most people regain all the weight they lost soon after stopping the pills. Clearly, these pills have many more risks than benefits. Furthermore, the side effects can be dangerous, including dehydration, coma, seizures, heart attacks, and even death.

What about Bariatric Surgery?

Bariatric surgery, commonly known as stomach-stapling, has been prominently featured in the news lately. Several high-profile individuals such as Al Roker and Star Jones have had the surgery. Medical television shows feature dramatic before-and-after photos of "everyday people" who have gone under the knife to lose weight.

This operation dramatically reduces the size of your stomach, so that you are unable to eat a large amount of food. By reducing the number of calories you consume, you lose weight. Obviously, this surgery is not for someone who is merely overweight. It is reserved for the very obese. As with any operation, there are serious risks associated with this procedure. If you think this option may be right for you, talk to your doctor.

THE BEST WAY TO LOSE WEIGHT AND KEEP IT OFF

Believe it or not, there is a 100 percent guaranteed way to lose weight and keep it off: eat less and move more. Eating a healthy diet and exercising every day is the best way to lose weight and improve your health at the same time.

1. *Make exercise a regular habit.* Work toward the goal of exercising thirty minutes a day most days of the week. Walking is one of the easiest and most effective forms of exercise, especially for beginners.

2. *Don't skip breakfast.* What you've heard about breakfast being the most important meal of the day is true. Starting your day with a healthy

breakfast revs up your metabolism and helps you burn calories more effectively all day. Skipping meals may seem to be a logical way to restrict calories and lose weight, but it makes no sense metabolically. When your body does not have a steady and constant supply of healthy food throughout the day, it goes into "starvation mode." This means that any calories you eat are stored as fat. Obviously, this is exactly the opposite of what needs to happen for weight loss. So, don't skip breakfast or any other meal for that matter. Yet what if you eat three meals a day but still feel hungry between meals? The temptation to eat unhealthy foods can sabotage your best-laid plans for weight loss. That's why my next tip is . . .

3. *Snack.* Yes, you read that right. Eating healthy snacks between meals keeps your blood sugar level and reduces the temptation to eat unhealthy foods. Try nuts, soup, baby carrots, or whole grain crackers with low-fat cheese. These snacks are filling, will take the edge off your hunger, and will remove the temptation to eat something more fattening. Once you've committed yourself to changing your eating and exercise habits, it's natural to have a strong desire to see the needle on the scale make a dramatic shift. But that's not the best strategy for lasting weight loss. In fact . . .

4. *Don't try to lose a large amount of weight overnight.* Although it's very tempting to try a diet that promises quick and dramatic weight loss, most people who lose weight too rapidly gain it back over time. If you lose weight gradually, say between one and two pounds per week, you are more likely to keep it off over the long term. And it's not as hard as you might think. One pound is equivalent to 3,500 calories, so to lose a pound a week, you need to eliminate only 500 calories from your diet every day. If you're like most people, you enjoy drinking soda. A twenty-ounce bottle of soda contains 250 calories, so by eliminating two sodas a day (or eliminating one soda and riding your bike for thirty minutes a day), you will lose one pound a week without much effort. To double your weight loss, try eliminating a fast-food adult meal of a burger, fries, and soft drink, which adds up to about 1,000 calories. While you're considering what to eat and not eat . . .

5. *Keep a food diary*. Writing down everything you eat may seem like a chore, but it is an effective way to lose more weight. In fact, black women who kept a food diary lost twice as much weight as women who didn't.[6] In addition to making you more aware of what you eat, a food diary can help you eat more sensible portion sizes. Use the guidelines in table 11 to gauge your portions.

Naturally, as you begin to adopt a healthier way of life in your mission to lose weight, you will want to continue to track your BMI. As you do so, I need to offer you a caution and a word of encouragement. It is entirely possible for you to exercise regularly, eat healthy foods, and find that your BMI is still in the overweight range. Don't worry. By eating right and exercising, you have lost weight and built muscle mass. Muscle weighs more than fat, which may be why your BMI is elevated. In addition, your ultimate size is determined in part by your genetics. This means that there are some physically active people who may never be thin by today's standards. Remember, a healthy weight is not defined by a dress or shirt size. You can be healthy in a wide range of sizes. We're not all meant to be thin. But we are all meant to be healthy! As long as your

Table 11. Sensible portion sizes

A single serving of . . .	Is the size of . . .
Meat or fish	Deck of cards
Rice or pasta	1/2 baseball
Salad greens or medium piece of fruit	1 baseball
Baked potato	Fist
Cereal	Fist
Cornbread	Bar of soap
Margarine	1 dice
Cheese	4 stacked dice or 2 slices
Ice cream	1/2 baseball

waist-hip ratio is less than 1.0, keep doing what you're doing. You're on the right track. Studies comparing the health of individuals who are "overweight" but fit with that of individuals who are thin but inactive show that it's healthier to be overweight and fit. Physical inactivity at any weight has a detrimental effect on your health.

LOSING WEIGHT REQUIRES SUPPORT

If you discover that you need to lose weight, seek support from family, friends, and even programs like Weight Watchers to help you stay on track. Support can also be found online. Websites like ediets.com provide an online community where people can share their weight-loss success stories and provide words of encouragement and wisdom that increase your likelihood of reaching your healthy weight. The reason many black women fail to meet their weight-loss goals is that they don't have adequate support. I have friends who have had the best of intentions to lose a few pounds, only to become quickly discouraged and give up after one setback. What they don't realize is that setbacks are a normal part of the long weight-loss process. It's hard to keep yourself motivated all the time. That's why it's so important not to go it alone.

If family members or friends need to lose weight, don't ridicule their intentions or try to talk them out of losing weight. Applaud their decision, and celebrate small accomplishments like the first pound lost, the first ten pounds lost, and so forth. Encourage your loved ones if they "fall off the wagon." We all miss the mark from time to time, but the most important thing is to get back up and keep moving toward the goal. Be there to talk your loved ones through the lows. Provide a listening ear when they become discouraged.

Be willing to change your habits to support your loved one. One reason black women have trouble losing weight and maintaining weight loss is that their family members refuse to eat healthier meals. Women often feel obligated to prepare foods preferred by family members and are then tempted to eat the less healthy meals. Instead of insisting on fried chicken, be willing to eat the baked chicken . . . without the skin! Furthermore, don't tempt or sabotage family members on a weight-loss program by eating a forbidden food in their presence or offering them a food they shouldn't eat.

THE ULTIMATE GOAL

Maintaining a healthy weight is *not* about going on a diet or taking a diet pill. It's about reaching a balance between the calories you eat and the calories you burn through physical activity. African Americans can no longer afford to be double-minded. Obesity is the number-one health problem in the black community, and we must become crystal clear and singularly focused on eliminating the health threat that it poses.

I like Web MD's definition of healthy weight: "A healthy weight is the weight your body naturally settles into when you consistently eat a nutritious diet, are physically active, and balance the calories you eat with the physical activity you do." This definition is great because it lists four criteria that define your healthy weight:

1. You *consistently* eat a nutritious diet.
2. You *consistently* exercise.
3. You *balance* your diet and your physical activity.
4. Your healthy weight is not a size, but is the weight your body *naturally* settles into when you begin to live a healthy lifestyle.

This means that your healthy weight is yours alone. It's individual. It's personal. And it's the result of a balanced way of living.

MORE FOOD FOR THOUGHT

1. Good self-esteem is important at any weight. But why is it dangerous to carry around extra weight, no matter how good you feel about yourself?

2. Think of a situation where a friend told you about her plans to lose weight. How did you handle it? Could you have handled it better? How would you handle the situation today?

3. Reflect on the differences between the way blacks and whites view weight. How are both viewpoints unhealthy?

4. What is obesity? Name three reasons why it is dangerous. How many black men are obese? How many black women are obese?

5. What is a calorie? Where do calories come from? Name the three factors that determine how many calories you need every day. What happens if you consume more calories than you need?

6. Why are most people with type 2 diabetes overweight?

7. Why is abdominal fat so dangerous?

8. Why don't starvation diets work? Why is it important not to allow yourself to get hungry when trying to lose weight?

9. Name three reasons why fad diets are unhealthy.

10. What are the two steps to losing weight and keeping it off?

11. Why is breakfast so important?

12. Reflect on Web MD's definition of a healthy weight. Do you believe it's worthwhile to achieve?

CHAPTER THREE

From Soul Food to Food for the Soul:
The Keys to Eating Well

I n our quest to improve African American health, we place too much emphasis on pharmaceutical treatments and medical procedures, when in fact we need look no further than our own plates. More than any pill or potion, healthy eating habits have the greatest potential to help African Americans stay well. A healthy diet can reduce your risk of obesity, high blood pressure, cancer, and heart disease. In fact, 14 percent of all premature deaths have been linked to what we eat.[1] Today's food choices today have a profound impact on tomorrow's quality of life. And the choice couldn't be clearer. Choose wisely and live a longer and healthier life. Choose poorly, and your chances of getting sick increase exponentially.

I'll be the first to admit that my diet has room for improvement. I could stand to drink more water, stay away from the fried foods, and just say no to dessert. And apparently, I'm not alone. According to the US Department of Agriculture, the diets of most Americans are not as healthy as they should be. When ranked for fruit and vegetables, fat, and fiber, 28 percent of African Americans', 16 percent of whites', and 14 percent of other racial and ethnic groups' diets were considered poor.[2] As a whole, African Americans tend to consume more meat, more saturated fat, more salt, and fewer fruits and vegetables than other racial and ethnic groups.

But food choice is not simply a matter of health for most African Americans. A clinical examination of how food influences health minimizes our joyful traditions of cooking and eating. We enjoy big meals served at big tables surrounded by happy people. For African Americans, food is more than nutrition and sustenance. Food is comfort after a long and difficult day on the job. Food is celebration—weddings, birthdays, graduations. Food is mourning—the black community brings food to the bereaved to say that we care. Food is socializing—family reunions and cookouts. Food is fellowship—church repasts provide a time to get to know one another. Food is a symbol of community and belonging. Black families across this country gather around the dinner table, the picnic table, and the banquet table to connect and feel at ease in a society that is not always comfortable. It is impossible to understand the symbolic meaning behind the traditional African American diet without understanding how our ways of cooking and eating have been shaped by our history.

HOG MEAT AND HOMINY

In the seventeenth, eighteenth, and nineteenth centuries, black slaves depended primarily on their masters for weekly rations of food—mostly pork scraps, salt, corn, and molasses. While white planters and slave owners and their families ate "high on the hog" (that is, the "better" parts of the hog), chicken, and cattle, they passed on to slaves their scraps—undesirable portions, including the feet, neck, ears, tail, intestine, kidneys, livers, and brains of the hog, and the feet, liver, and gizzards of chickens. Black female slaves seasoned the naturally bland pig feet, ham hocks, chitterlings, and pig ears with onions, garlic, bay leaves, and other herbs and spices to make them more flavorful. Slaves also received an allotment of salt, which was used not only as a seasoning but also as a preservative. Salt pork and fatback—remnants of pork scraps preserved in salt brine—seasoned greens and other vegetables that the cooks scraped together. Cornbread, made from cornmeal mixed with water, "meat," and occasional vegetables formed the core of most slave meals. Molasses was used as a sweetener or mixed with bacon grease to make a "sap" that slaves ate with cornbread.[3]

Not much changed for blacks after emancipation. In fact, for the mostly uneducated, illiterate (reading was illegal for slaves), and impoverished former slaves, freedom was more conceptual than real. To say that employment opportunities for former slaves were limited is an understatement. Sharecropping and tenant farming were the only forms of employment available to most southern African Americans. Most sharecroppers subsisted on a pork- and corn-based (hog meat and hominy) diet, not unlike the foods eaten by slaves, because these foods were relatively plentiful and cheap. Even former slaves who migrated west and north maintained these ways of cooking as a reminder of the familiar tastes and comforts of home and family amid unfamiliar surroundings.

From Slave Food to Soul Food

Southern blacks continued the practice of passing down recipes through the generations, preserving long-standing eating practices. This way of cooking and eating gained a stronger foothold and a new name—soul food—in the 1960s during the black power movement. Soul food documented our troubled history and symbolized our triumph in the most evil of circumstances: slavery. Soul food celebrates and preserves our unique ethnic identity and is a symbol of our cultural pride and unity.

Symbolism aside, the harsh reality is that soul food's core ingredients, some combination of fat, salt, and sugar, contribute to our sky-high rates of disease (table 12).

Tradition is not the only factor keeping us from eating healthier. Time, or lack thereof, is also to blame. Eating on the run has become a way of life for most American families—including black families. Rush-

Table 12. Diet-related disease by race and gender (percent of population)

	Obesity	Diabetes	High blood pressure
Blacks			
Male	21.1	7.6	36.7
Female	37.4	11.2	36.6
Total	33.4	10.8	36.6
Whites			
Male	20.0	4.7	24.6
Female	22.4	5.4	20.5
Total	21.3	7.8	22.1
Hispanics			
Male	23.1	8.1	N/A
Female	33.0	11.4	N/A
Total	26.2	9.0	N/A

Source: CDC/NCHS 2002.

ing to get dinner on the table between work, football practice, and choir rehearsal leaves little time to prepare meals from scratch. And in our overworked, under-rested lives, we have too much on our plates to worry about what's on our plates. That's why fast foods and convenience foods have become so popular over recent years. Although these foods may be quick to prepare or purchase, they often contain the same core ingredients as soul food—fat, salt, and sugar. Furthermore, they are full of calories and often empty of essential nutrients. Consider the typical diet of one of my adolescent patients—a fast-food breakfast sandwich in the morning, a fast-food "chicken box" for lunch, and Chinese take-out for dinner (table 13).

Table 13. Typical fast-food diet

	Calories	Saturated fat (g)	Sodium (mg)
Breakfast			
Ham, egg, and English muffin sandwich	300	5	820
Hash browns	150	1.5	310
Orange juice	140	0	5
Lunch			
Chicken (2 pieces dark meat)	220	3	620
Large potato wedges	260	2.5	740
Biscuit	180	2	540
Large soda	310	0	20
Dinner			
Egg rolls (2)	400	4	800
Shrimp lo mein	1,100	7	350
Large soda	300	0	20
Total	3,360	25	4,225

My patient ate three relatively inexpensive, filling, and tasty meals. But he got more than he bargained for because he actually consumed one and a half days' worth of calories (considering that the average adult requires about 2,000 calories a day), almost two days' worth of sodium (three days' worth if you are on a salt-restricted diet for high blood pressure), and more than a day's worth of saturated fat (recommended intake is no more than 15 to 20 grams a day).

The problem is that although most people have heard of the link between food and disease, they don't quite understand it. How can the food we eat cause some of the most deadly conditions of our day?

Your Diet and Your Health

Two landmark long-term studies followed adults for several decades, recording what they ate, what they drank, whether they exercised, and their overall health. These studies, the Framingham Study and the Nurses Health Study, are responsible for thousands of scientific discoveries about the relationship between our eating patterns and our health. Because of these studies, we understand that LDL cholesterol is linked to heart disease and that red meat increases the risk of cancer.

HOW FOOD CAUSES DISEASE

To understand how these foods can be so harmful, you need to know a bit about what happens when you eat. During the process of digestion, food is broken down into sugar, fatty acids, and amino acids. These substances are absorbed into the bloodstream and transported to cells, where they are converted into energy in a metabolic process called oxidation. Just as your car burns gas to produce energy, your body burns food (in the presence of oxygen) to produce energy. This energy is used to maintain all of your bodily functions.

A by-product of this process is the production of free radicals, unstable molecules that damage blood vessels, cells, tissues, and organs (fig. 4). Think of the process this way: when you burn wood in a fireplace, small embers are often thrown off. In the same way, when your food is digested to produce energy, free radicals are thrown off. Your body has its own internal sprinkler system that douses these free radicals before they can do any damage. But certain foods produce more free radicals than your body can handle. These foods tend to be highly processed, easily digested, and quickly absorbed in the bloodstream. This may not sound so bad, but their quick absorption means that instead of your cells producing a steady flow of energy, they produce an explosion of energy all at once. This overload of energy generates excessive free radicals that overwhelm your body's internal sprinkler system. By regularly eating the wrong types of foods, your body consistently pumps out excess free radi-

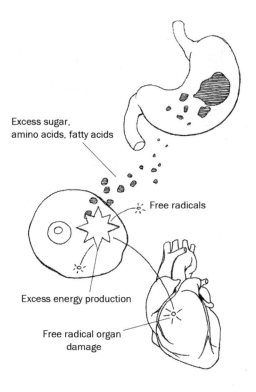

Figure 4. How overeating causes free radical organ damage.

cals. Returning to the previous example, when you burn wood in a fireplace, some sparking embers can land on the carpet and leave small burn holes. In the same way, excess free radicals "land" on the cells in your body and cause organ damage that ultimately results in heart disease, stroke, diabetes, and cancer. Which foods cause this persistent surplus of free radicals? Foods that contain sugar, saturated and trans fats, and processed carbohydrates.[4]

Sugar

Baked goods like cakes, pies, and cookies and sweetened drinks like soda, Kool-Aid, and sweet tea are high in "empty calories," meaning that the sugar in these foods increases their calorie content but adds little nutritional value. Here's what I mean. A typical twenty-ounce soda contains 250 calories (from about fifteen teaspoons of sugar) and provides no vitamins, minerals, or other important nutrients (empty calories). A sweet tooth is not only harmful to your waistline and your teeth; it also threatens your heart health. Sugar from these foods is easily digested and absorbed into your bloodstream, setting the stage for excess free radical production and organ damage. A better choice to satisfy your sugar craving is fruit. Although fruit contains sugar, it also contains vitamins, minerals, and fiber that, when digested, slow the absorption of sugar into your bloodstream and prevent the overproduction of free radicals.

Saturated and Trans Fats

In addition to increasing your body's production of free radicals, saturated fats increase your risk of heart attack by raising the levels of LDL (bad) cholesterol that tends to accumulate in the blood vessels surrounding your heart. These artery-clogging fats are solid at room temperature and are found in animal products such as red meat, chicken (especially the skin), ribs, chitterlings, pig's feet, butter, cheese, whole milk, sausage, and bacon. (Note that ham hocks, chitterlings, pig's feet, neck bones, salt pork, and fatback are not considered to be meat. They are mostly saturated fat.) Frying chicken, steak, okra, green tomatoes, and fish in shortening or lard, a practice that hearkens back to our West African roots, adds even more saturated fat. Most home-style gravy—a delicious blend of flour and meat drippings—is also high in fat. Saturated fat can even be found in collard greens, peas, and beans that have been cooked with ham hocks, salt pork, or fatback. Yet another source of saturated fat could be found in an aluminum can on the stoves in most black households when I was a child. It may be on top of your stove right now. This can stored bacon grease, which would be used when cooking food like cornbread or scrambled eggs. Bacon grease is very high in saturated fat and should not be used for cooking.

Trans fats are artificially created and are found in snack cakes, cookies, and crackers, frozen fish sticks and pizzas, fast-food fried chicken and french fries, and other "junk" foods. Like saturated fats, trans fats increase your risk of heart disease by increasing free radicals and raising levels of LDL (bad) cholesterol; they also lower levels of HDL (good) cholesterol. They are the worst fats for your blood vessels and heart health and should be avoided altogether. Check your food labels for "partially hydrogenated vegetable oil," another term for trans fats. New York City has banned the use of trans fats, and other cities and states are considering doing the same.

Processed Carbohydrates

The popularity of low-carb diets has led many people to believe that carbs are bad and make you fat. This couldn't be further from the truth. Carbohydrates, found in foods such as breads, grains, pasta, rice, fruits, and vegetables, are an essential part of a balanced diet. The problem is that many carbohydrates found in convenience foods are processed into an easily digestible food that rapidly raises blood sugar and increases free radical production. For example, white flour is made by removing the outer layers of fiber and bran from whole wheat fiber. Processed carbohydrates like white bread, white rice, and white pasta (such as macaroni and spaghetti) also add excess calories while providing few to no necessary nutrients. Whole-grain breads and pastas and brown rice are healthier choices. Another tip: when buying bread or crackers, don't just trust the name. For example, a lot of bread sold as "wheat bread" is actually made from processed flour. Check the ingredients list on the label. If it lists "enriched" flour, don't buy it . . . it's not whole grain.

Salt

Although not directly implicated in free radical production, salt is a significant cause of disease for African Americans. Salt causes water retention, which raises blood pressure. Because blacks tend to be more sensitive to the effects of salt, it raises our blood pressure even higher than that of whites. Most of us eat more salt than we realize. Thanks to our preference for highly seasoned foods, we tend to add salt during cooking. In addition, salt, in the form of sodium, is a practically universal ingredient hidden in canned, packaged, and restaurant foods. Remember, the recommended daily salt intake should not exceed 2,300 mg sodium. Check food labels carefully.

WE MUST EAT HEALTHIER

The USDA Healthy Eating Index scored the average diet of African Americans as highest in total fat, saturated fat, and salt. Our diets scored lowest in consumption of fruits, vegetables, and whole grains.[5] According to the *American Journal of Preventive Medicine,* only 7 percent of African Americans meet the recommended guidelines of five to nine servings of fruits and vegetables per day. The facts are clear—our ways of cooking and eating raise our risk of disease. Therefore it stands to reason that we must modify our diet to improve our health.

For those who enjoy eating traditional African American meals, I know that I am treading on dangerous ground. Don't get me wrong. I am not saying that all traditional foods are unhealthy. In fact, vegetables like collard greens, cabbage, turnips, sweet potatoes, and kale contain essential vitamins and minerals, are naturally low in fat and sugar, and contain no cholesterol (table 14). Fresh peas and beans are a good source of fiber. But remember, cooking these vegetables in ham hocks, salt pork, or fatback counteracts the healthful benefits.

I also acknowledge that not all African Americans eat traditional foods. But many of us do. If you need proof, travel to any black neighborhood in any major city in this country and you'll find a soul food restaurant. From elaborate dining halls to hole-in-the-wall joints, these restaurants do a brisk business from those of us who enjoy our traditional meals. Furthermore, traditional foods are featured prominently at such special events and occasions as holidays, church repasts, and other celebrations.

You may think, "Our ancestors ate this way and were healthy. Why

Table 14. Healthy soul food

Healthy soul food	Contains . . .	Protects you from . . .
Black-eyed peas, red beans, black beans	Fiber and antioxidants	Cancer and heart disease
Kale, collard greens, mustard greens	Lutein	Cataracts
Sweet potatoes	Beta carotene (source of Vitamin A)	Vision problems
Tomatoes	Lycopene	Cancer
Okra	Potassium	High blood pressure

can't we eat the same way?" But there are three major differences between the way our ancestors ate and the way we eat today.

First, our ancestors ate smaller portions. Slaves were given small weekly rations of food for their family. The portions of food we eat are much larger. In fact, over the past twenty years, portion sizes have grown dramatically, according to the National Heart, Lung, and Blood Institute. A fast-food cheeseburger that was 333 calories has now grown to 590 calories. A small order of french fries that was once 2.4 ounces and 210 calories has now inflated to 6.9 ounces and 610 calories. And a soda that was 6.5 ounces and 85 calories is now 20 ounces and 250 calories. Put into another context, consider a typical plate of food at a large family dinner or church repast: two pieces of fried chicken, two slices of ham, mashed potatoes and gravy, dressing (stuffing), string beans, greens, a dinner roll with butter, a scoop of macaroni and cheese, a serving of peach cobbler, and a 20-ounce soft drink. This one plate contains more than 1,900 calories—the total number of calories that should be eaten by most adults in a single day!

Second, our ancestors were more active. Slave work was hard manual labor. Slaves worked from sunup to sundown, and they easily burned every calorie they ate. Most of today's jobs don't require us to work nearly as hard; modern conveniences like computers, remote controls, elevators, and automobiles have made all Americans a very sedentary people. This lack of physical activity means that most of the calories we eat are not burned but stored as fat.

Third, our ancestors' food was mainly "organic," while many of the foods we eat are processed. The meat our ancestors ate was freshly slaughtered, and vegetables went directly from the garden to the table. Today, much of the meat we eat has been treated with antibiotics or steroids, and fruits and vegetables have been treated with pesticides. Packaged meats, fruits, and vegetables have been treated with added salt and other chemicals that prolong shelf life but diminish their nutritional value.

Ultimately, it doesn't matter whether you eat traditional African American meals or the "modern" Western diet of packaged, processed, and fast foods. If we continue to regularly consume animal fat, then we will continue to die from heart disease at a greater rate than whites. If we continue to eat salty foods, then our position atop the world's ranking for high blood pressure will remain secure. If we continue to choose sweet snacks and drinks, we will remain the most obese group in the nation.

GIVE YOUR DIET A MAKEOVER

Now that you have committed to making your soul food healthier, what about the rest of your diet? There is no shortage of nutrition advice, and it ranges from the reasonable to the ridiculous. Good eating habits are not complicated and don't require starvation or deprivation. I will share several tips on how to improve your diet with minimal pain and effort, and you'll be pleasantly surprised to learn that rather than telling you what *not* to eat, these tips (with one exception) tell you what *to* eat.

Following these tips is important, but cut yourself some slack if you occasionally slip up. While some of your favorite foods may be less healthy, indulging in them every now and then is not the end of the world. The most important thing to remember is balance. For example, if

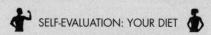 SELF-EVALUATION: YOUR DIET

Is it time to make a few changes in your diet? Respond to each statement using the following scale:

5 = always   4 = often   3 = sometimes   2 = rarely   1 = never

1. ___ I eat fast food or carryout foods three or more times a week.
2. ___ I drink sweet tea or soda with every meal.
3. ___ I cook my vegetables with fatback, salt pork, or ham hocks.
4. ___ I shake salt on all my food before I taste it.
5. ___ I must have something sweet (such as cake, cookies, pie, or ice cream) at the end of my meals.
6. ___ I keep a can of bacon grease on my stove.

How's your current diet? A score of 6 means that your diet lowers your risk of illness, and probably protects you from getting sick. If your score is closer to 30, here are three ways to make your soul food healthier:

1. Bake or broil instead of fry.
2. Rather than ordering out, cook your own food and season it with herbs, spices, garlic, and onion instead of salt.
3. Reduce the amount of pork fat (chitterlings, ham hocks, salt pork, pig's ears, fatback) that you eat. These are not "everyday" foods, so save them for special occasions.

Several cookbooks show you how to make healthier substitutions for the salt and fat used in traditional soul food recipes, while preserving the flavor of down-home cooking. Fabiola Demps Gaines and Roniece Weaver's *New Soul Food Cookbook for People with Diabetes* (Alexandria, VA: American Diabetes Association, 2006) gets this southern girl's seal of approval . . . and it's not just for people with diabetes.

FROM SOUL FOOD TO FOOD FOR THE SOUL

you eat a lunch of fried chicken wings, fries, and a soda, balance it with a dinner of baked fish, salad, and a glass of water. Pay attention to what you eat throughout the day to make sure that your overall diet contains mostly nutritious and healthy choices.

SIX STEPS TO EATING RIGHT

1. *Add more color to your meals.* Look at your plate. What color is your food? Constantly eating meals in shades of brown and beige—for example, a meal of fried chicken, mashed potatoes and gravy, and a roll—won't provide you with the proper balance of nutrients to keep you in optimal health. Adding a shot of color to every meal is what the doctor ordered to make your food work for you. One of the easiest ways to improve your diet is to eat more fruits and vegetables of every color. Try red strawberries, apples, and cherries; orange carrots, sweet potatoes, and tangerines; yellow squash and pineapples; green peppers, broccoli, kale, spinach, lettuce, and honeydews; purple grapes and plums; blueberries; and white cauliflower, corn, and peaches. Here are three key reasons why eating fruits and vegetables is so important.

- Fruits and vegetables keep you well. Because they are naturally low in fat, sodium, and cholesterol, eating five servings of fruits and vegetables a day helps you prevent high blood pressure, coronary heart disease, stroke, and diabetes.[6]
- Fruits and vegetables help you manage your weight. They are naturally low in calories and high in fiber. Therefore, they fill you up while reducing your total caloric intake. They make a convenient and healthy snack that can stave off the hunger pangs that usually tempt you to reach for potato chips or candy. The fiber they contain helps detoxify your body by sweeping waste out of your colon; think of it as an all-natural colon cleanser.
- Fruits and vegetables fight cancer and aging. Fruits and vegetables contain phytochemicals—substances that fight disease by

preventing the inflammatory cellular damage caused by free radicals. The more colorful your choices, the greater health benefits for you.

Eating just five servings of fruits and vegetables a day has been proven to lower the risk of illness. Although five servings may sound like a lot, they can be easily spread over your daily food intake if you include fruits and vegetables in your breakfast, lunch, dinner, and snacks. You'll be surprised how easy it is to incorporate five servings into your day. If you eat a sliced banana in a bowl of cereal for breakfast, a large salad for lunch, an apple for snack, and a serving of greens for dinner with a bowl of sliced fruit for dessert, you've hit your mark. As a reference, one serving of a fruit or vegetable equals half a cup of cooked leafy vegetables (such as greens or spinach), half a cup of raw nonleafy vegetables, cut-up fruit, or fruit juice, or one medium piece of whole fruit.

If you're still not convinced of the power of adding fruits and vegetables to your diet, consider the following information. A Harvard School of Public Health study showed that eating five servings of fruits and vegetables a day lowered the risk of stroke by 30 percent. A reduced risk of stroke was detected starting at just three servings per day, but the maximum protection was seen at five servings per day of kale, broccoli, cauliflower, cabbage, collards, brussels sprouts, spinach, or grapefruit. A newer scientific study adds to our knowledge that broccoli in particular is a superfood. This study showed that eating broccoli can undo the internal damage caused by high blood sugar. This means that diabetics can reduce their risk of heart disease, blindness, kidney disease, and amputations by eating broccoli. More research is needed to confirm this finding, but consider this another good reason to eat your veggies.[7]

Fresh fruits and vegetables are best, but frozen produce is another healthy and affordable option. If you eat canned vegetables, choose low-salt or no-salt options. When these are not available, discard the liquid from the can and rinse the vegetables before cooking. Make sure canned fruits are packed in juice—not syrup—and have little or no added sugar.

No special preparation is required to enjoy the considerable health benefits of these wonder foods. You can eat them raw, steamed, and in salads and soups. Don't throw away the water you cook them in, because your grandmother was right. The pot liquor is full of vitamins and nutrients. Also, remember to season with garlic, onion, bell pepper, and spices instead of salt and pork fat.

One final point: as I speak to audiences across the country, I frequently hear the complaint that "healthy foods" like fresh fruits and vegetables are expensive. Although I can't deny that a fast-food meal may be less expensive than buying a bunch of grapes, apples, and red bell peppers, in the long run the cost of eating healthier pales in comparison to the billions of dollars you and I spend each year treating disease in our community. Doesn't it make more sense to invest our earnings in our well-being instead of continuing to dissipate our hard-earned dollars in an attempt to regain our health?

2. *Eat fish twice a week.* Certain fish—salmon, herring, lake trout, mackerel, and sardines—are high in omega-3 fatty acids (table 15). Also known as fish oils, omega-3 fatty acids are healthy fats that are good for your heart. They prevent heart disease, lower triglycerides, prevent a second heart attack, and slightly lower blood pressure. Omega-3's also reduce inflammation and slow the progression of atherosclerosis (hardening of the arteries) in patients with heart disease. Baking or broiling fish is healthier than frying. Fish may also be sautéed in olive oil.

If you don't like fish, over-the-counter omega-3 supplements are also effective. Look for fish oil supplements that provide a total of 1,000 mg DHA and EPA (two types of omega-3 fatty acids; check the labels). Check with your doctor before taking fish oil supplements if you are allergic to fish, if you take blood thinners, or if you are pregnant or have a medical condition.

3. *Shake the salt habit.* The American Heart Association recommends that we consume no more than one teaspoon of salt a day (2,300 mg of sodium). But the average American consumes at least three times as much salt, a level of consumption that is unhealthy for all Americans,

Table 15. Recommended omega-3 intakes

Health condition	Recommendation
If you do not have coronary heart disease	Eat fish twice a week. Walnuts are also high in omega-3 fats; eat about a handful a day. (Other medical sources also suggest taking 1,000 mg fish oil supplements once a day.)
If you have been diagnosed with coronary heart disease	Eat fish every day. Because heart disease patients may not be able to get enough omega-3 fats through diet alone, consider taking 1,000 mg fish oil supplements daily. Ask your doctor.
If you have high blood triglyceride (fat) levels	Higher doses (2,000–4,000 mg a day) of omega-3 fats are needed to lower triglyceride levels. This dosage must be taken under a doctor's care.

Source: Adapted from http://www.americanheart.org/presenter.jhtml?identifier=4632.

but is especially problematic for blacks because we are more sensitive to salt's negative effects on blood pressure. According to the National Heart, Lung, and Blood Institute, cutting sodium intake by half would prevent 150,000 deaths from heart disease each year. You may assume that removing the salt shaker from the dinner table will significantly reduce your intake, but you'd be wrong. Most dietary salt (in the form of sodium) comes from processed foods like canned soups, boxed cereals, snack foods, hot dogs, lunch meats, soy sauce, and bouillon cubes. You can reduce your daily salt intake by up to 40 percent just by removing one high-salt food. Read nutrition labels; try to make sure each serving you eat contains less than 5 percent of the FDA recommended daily value for sodium.

4. *Detoxify your system.* Brown rice, fresh fruits and vegetables, and whole grain breads and cereals provide fiber, a natural detoxifier that sweeps the waste out of your colon and helps prevent colon cancer. Fiber is a great way to control your weight because it prevents overeating by making you feel full. It also lowers "bad" LDL cholesterol which reduces the risk of heart disease, and prevents constipation by causing regular bowel movements. According to the Harvard School of Public Health, most adults should eat at least twenty grams of fiber a day, and more is better.[8] Check nutrition labels—any food with five or more grams of fiber is considered to be a high fiber food.

5. *Take a multivitamin.* Although a balanced diet will provide you with all of the nutrients your body needs, only 10 percent of Americans eat a diet that meets all nutrition recommendations.[9] That's why the rest of us need to take a daily multivitamin. Most general daily vitamins on the market contain sufficient doses of essential nutrients to meet your needs. The only exception is vitamin D—if your multivitamin doesn't provide 1,000 IU, you should take a supplement to get you up to the desired level. A final caution: don't take mega-doses of vitamins.

With the abundance of food in this country, it is probably hard for you to imagine that anyone would be malnourished. But nutritional deficiencies are not limited to countries with an insufficient food supply. It is possible to overeat and still fall short of the recommended daily intake of nutrients because fast foods, soft drinks, snack foods, and alcoholic beverages are full of calories, but contain few to no nutrients. In fact, most nutritionists agree that the average American is deficient in several nutrients; three deficiencies are a particular problem for African Americans—calcium, vitamin D, and potassium.

- Calcium: Although blacks are less likely to be diagnosed with osteoporosis (weak bones), we are still at risk because we don't get sufficient calcium in our diets—50 percent less than recommended according to the National Institutes of Health. We should get around 1,000 mg calcium per day, but our lactose intolerance—an estimated

75 percent of African Americans have this condition—means that we don't benefit from the calcium found in dairy products. There are, however, other good sources of calcium. For example, one cup of cooked collard greens has more calcium than one cup of milk. Other green leafy vegetables like spinach, kale, and turnip greens are good sources of calcium, as are canned sardines and salmon (with the bones) and fortified cereals and juices.[10]

- Vitamin D: Vitamin D deficiency occurs in people who do not get enough sunlight. Our dark skin contains melanin, a natural sunscreen that blocks our ability to make sufficient vitamin D (a process initiated by the skin's exposure to sunlight). Very few foods naturally contain vitamin D; milk and cereal are fortified with the vitamin. If you're lactose intolerant, take a supplement that provides 1,000 IU vitamin D per day.

- Potassium: Potassium helps you keep your blood pressure in check by balancing the amount of sodium (salt) in your body.[11] As a result, diets rich in potassium lower your blood pressure. You should have no problem reaching the recommended 4,700 mg potassium per day by eating plenty of fruits and vegetables, including such foods as sweet potatoes, avocados, lima beans, orange juice, bananas, and apricots.

6. *Read nutrition labels.* When the government devised food labels, it certainly seemed like a good idea . . . to help us figure out if a packaged food is worth eating. The problem is that these labels, like most government documents, are almost impossible to decipher. What are "percent daily values"? How do you interpret serving sizes? Yet all government put-downs aside, food labels serve an important purpose by allowing you to weigh the relative nutritive value of one packaged food against another so that you can make smart choices for you and your family. Follow these simple steps to make reading nutrition labels—and choosing healthier foods—easier. More detailed instructions can be found in Frequently Asked Questions, at the back of this book.

Figure 5. How to read a food label.

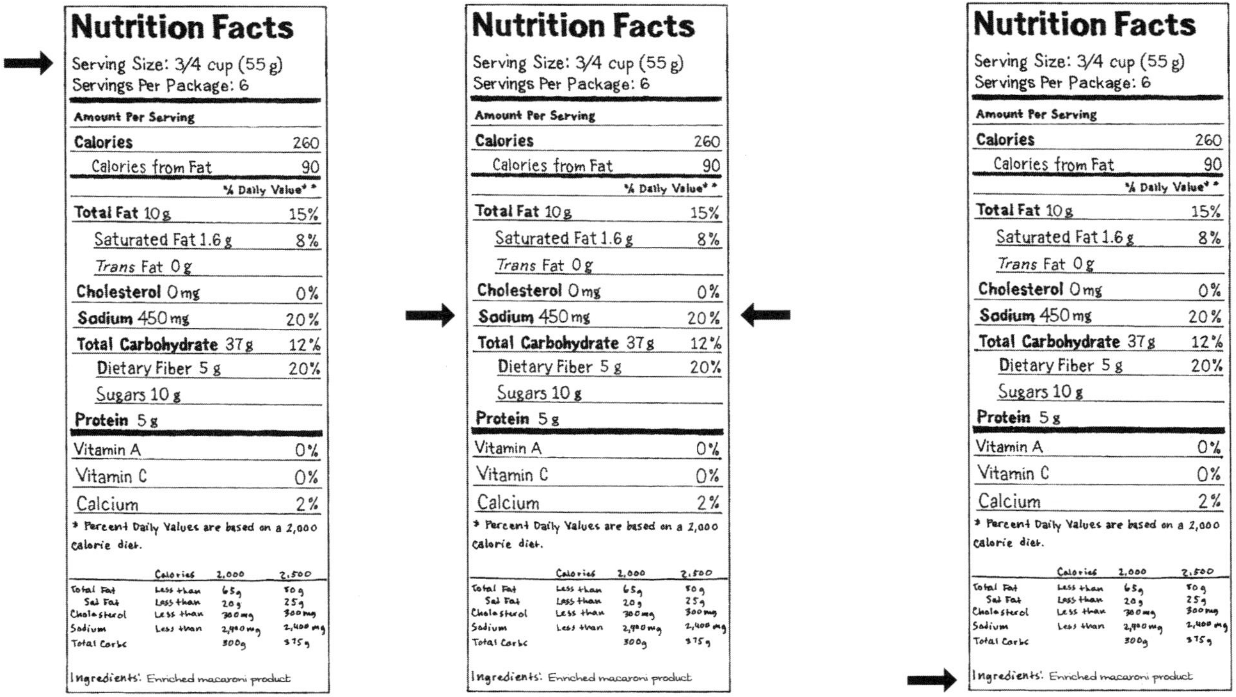

(a)

Nutrition Facts

Serving Size: 3/4 cup (55 g)
Servings Per Package: 6

Amount Per Serving

Calories	260
Calories from Fat	90

% Daily Value *

Total Fat 10 g	15%
Saturated Fat 1.6 g	8%
Trans Fat 0 g	
Cholesterol 0 mg	0%
Sodium 450 mg	20%
Total Carbohydrate 37 g	12%
Dietary Fiber 5 g	20%
Sugars 10 g	
Protein 5 g	
Vitamin A	0%
Vitamin C	0%
Calcium	2%

* Percent Daily Values are based on a 2,000 Calorie diet.

	Calories	2,000	2,500
Total Fat	Less than	65 g	80 g
Sat Fat	Less than	20 g	25 g
Cholesterol	Less than	300 mg	300 mg
Sodium	Less than	2,400 mg	2,400 mg
Total Carbs		300 g	375 g

Ingredients: Enriched macaroni product.

(a) First, check the serving size.

(b)

Nutrition Facts

Serving Size: 3/4 cup (55 g)
Servings Per Package: 6

Amount Per Serving

Calories	260
Calories from Fat	90

% Daily Value *

Total Fat 10 g	15%
Saturated Fat 1.6 g	8%
Trans Fat 0 g	
Cholesterol 0 mg	0%
Sodium 450 mg	20%
Total Carbohydrate 37 g	12%
Dietary Fiber 5 g	20%
Sugars 10 g	
Protein 5 g	
Vitamin A	0%
Vitamin C	0%
Calcium	2%

* Percent Daily Values are based on a 2,000 Calorie diet.

	Calories	2,000	2,500
Total Fat	Less than	65 g	80 g
Sat Fat	Less than	20 g	25 g
Cholesterol	Less than	300 mg	300 mg
Sodium	Less than	2,400 mg	2,400 mg
Total Carbs		300 g	375 g

Ingredients: Enriched macaroni product.

(b) Next, look at the nutrients section. This food is high in sodium.

(c)

Nutrition Facts

Serving Size: 3/4 cup (55 g)
Servings Per Package: 6

Amount Per Serving

Calories	260
Calories from Fat	90

% Daily Value *

Total Fat 10 g	15%
Saturated Fat 1.6 g	8%
Trans Fat 0 g	
Cholesterol 0 mg	0%
Sodium 450 mg	20%
Total Carbohydrate 37 g	12%
Dietary Fiber 5 g	20%
Sugars 10 g	
Protein 5 g	
Vitamin A	0%
Vitamin C	0%
Calcium	2%

* Percent Daily Values are based on a 2,000 Calorie diet.

	Calories	2,000	2,500
Total Fat	Less than	65 g	80 g
Sat Fat	Less than	20 g	25 g
Cholesterol	Less than	300 mg	300 mg
Sodium	Less than	2,400 mg	2,400 mg
Total Carbs		300 g	375 g

Ingredients: Enriched macaroni product.

(c) Finally, look at the ingredients list. This food's first ingredient is "enriched macaroni product," a processed carbohydrate.

- First, check the serving size (fig. 5a). The caloric and nutritional information is all based on a single serving size. If you plan to eat two servings, you need to double the calories and percent daily value.
- Next, look at the nutrients section (fig. 5b). Pay particular attention to the percent daily value column. Simply put, a percent daily value of 5 or lower means that the food is low in that nutrient. A percent daily value of 20 or higher means that the food is high in that nutrient. So if you have high blood pressure, you want to choose a low-salt food. The best choice for you is a food with less than or equal to 5 percent of your daily value of sodium per serving.
- Last, look at the ingredients list (fig. 5c). The shorter the list, the better. Ingredients are listed in order of weight (or amount) from most to least. This provides another useful way to choose healthy foods. For example, if you are trying to limit sugar in your diet, choose a food that does *not* have an added sugar as one of the first few ingredients. Also, look for the following repeat offenders found in less healthy foods: "high fructose corn syrup" (a sweetener), "partially hydrogenated vegetable oil" (a trans fat), and "enriched flour" (a processed carbohydrate).

A BETTER CHOICE

For people who arrived on these shores bereft of assets and stripped of culture, African Americans have created a proud legacy of foodways that has been passed down for nearly four hundred years from slavery to the present and one that demonstrates an ability to make something out of nothing. This legacy gives us strength. Soul food tells the story of how our ancestors came to this country and what happened when they got here. Nevertheless, although food provides a way to understand and honor our history, we must not maintain historical practices that are a clear threat to our health. As slaves, we had no choice but to eat what was provided for us. Today we have a choice. Let's proudly choose to pass on our traditions to future generations in a healthier way.

MORE FOOD FOR THOUGHT

1. Think about your diet. What are the best parts? Are there any changes that can make it healthier?

2. Review the three ways to make soul food healthier. Which are you willing to try?

3. Match the food items on the left with the diseases they are linked to. You can select the diseases more than once.

   a. salt   heart disease

   b. saturated fat   cancer

   c. trans fat   diabetes

   d. sugar   high blood pressure

4. Match the foods on the left with the diseases they help prevent. You can select the diseases more than once.

   a. okra   heart disease

   b. peaches   cancer

   c. salmon   stroke

   d. black-eyed peas   diabetes

   e. whole wheat bread   high blood pressure

5. Which diet-related diseases are more common in African Americans?

6. How can a nutrition label help you tell whether a food is low or high in calories? Low or high in sodium (salt)?

7. In which situations are you most tempted to eat a less healthy diet (for example, Thanksgiving dinner, family reunion, church repast)? Which of the following tips will be most helpful for you the next time you're in that situation?

   a. Eat a healthy snack (for example, a handful of nuts, baby carrots, an apple) before the big meal so you'll be less hungry.

   b. Drink a glass of water before eating.

   c. If soup or salad is served, eat that first to cut your appetite.

continued . . .

d. If both salad and dinner plates are available, use the salad plate for your dinner.

e. Load half your plate with vegetables, one fourth of your plate with a starch (rice, potatoes, bread), and the remaining fourth with meat.

f. Avoid gravies, sauces, and fried foods. If this is impossible, get only a small amount.

g. Split a dessert with a friend.

h. Drink water or diet soda with your meal.

CHAPTER FOUR

Make the Right Moves:
How to Burn Fat and Be Fit

African Americans have a long history of physical work. The United States was built by the sweat and backbreaking labor of our ancestors. The prosperity that our nation enjoys is directly proportional to the physical exertion put forth by millions of black slaves. After emancipation, the heavily agricultural economy provided our forefathers with plenty of work requiring manual labor. Our foremothers' housework was not assisted by power vacuums, electric washing machines, or cordless irons. More recently, we had to lift the garage door manually, get off the couch to change the television channel, and push our lawn mowers without the help of power-assist. We walked to school, church, and the store. In the past, getting enough physical activity was practically effortless. From the seventeenth century until modern times, African Americans have been fully acquainted with physical work.

That is why, until about a generation ago, getting adequate physical activity was not a major problem for blacks. But the past couple of decades have brought a dramatic shift in both the way we live and the way we make a living. Modern conveniences require much less physical exertion from us than was required of our parents and grandparents. Between the car, the computer, and the couch, many of us spend up to fifteen hours a day immobile! I know this from personal experience. I can spend my entire day sitting. I sit in traffic on the Beltway, in front of a computer, while talking on the phone, and in meeting after meeting. At the end of the day, I sit and hold my throbbing head! I am mentally and physically drained. My head hurts, my eyes are red, and my neck is stiff.

Now that physical activity is no longer a part of our daily routine, we have to schedule time to exercise. Some people choose to exercise before work in the morning; others like to exercise after work. But many others skip physical activity altogether, and it's not hard to imagine why. With so many obligations—job, family, hobbies, social activities—finding the spare time for physical activity often seems impossible. At the end of the workday, many people are so worn out that they have absolutely no motivation to work out.

WHAT IS PHYSICAL ACTIVITY AND WHY IS IT SO IMPORTANT?

Any action that involves motion (that is, the contraction of skeletal muscles) and boosts metabolism (thereby burning calories) is a physical activity. Walking, dancing, climbing stairs, raking leaves, playing basketball, cutting logs, lifting boxes, and participating in aerobics classes are examples of physical activity. The term "exercise" is often used interchangeably with physical activity (as I do in this chapter); technically, exercise is a more structured form of physical activity. There are three main categories of exercise—strength training, flexibility training, and aerobic exercise (fig. 6). Strength training and flexibility training build strong muscles and bones, improve mobility, and reduce the risk of injury from falls. Aerobic exercise has been proven to improve the health and function of your heart, lungs, and circulatory system and to reduce the risk of disease and premature death.

The health benefits of exercise increase in what scientists call a dose-response fashion. This is good news because it means that the more you

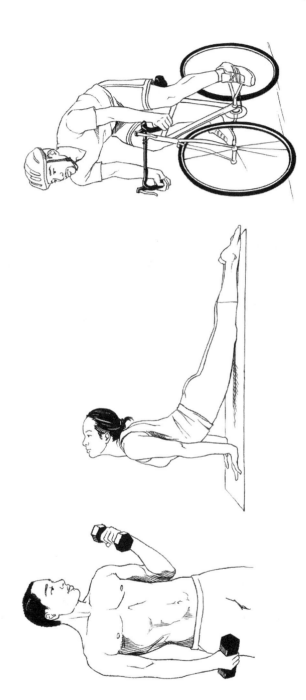

Figure 6. From left: strength, flexibility, and aerobic exercise.

exercise, the more benefits you realize. You don't need to be a serious athlete or even join a gym or participate in exercise classes to gain positive results. In fact, you will begin to reap the benefits of exercise with fairly minimal effort.

You needn't know the precise physiological terms and meanings of exercise in order to begin to enjoy its benefits. The most important things to remember are: (1) physical activity wards off disease, (2) physical activity prolongs your life, and (3) any amount is beneficial.

Despite these compelling facts, about 60 percent of adults don't do enough physical activity to get any health benefit. On average, women are less active than men, and African Americans are less active than whites. Black women, whose roles as caretakers of the family require them to juggle multiple responsibilities every day, are the least physically active of all groups. This means that among their many competing priorities at work, home, and community, scheduling time for physical activity usually loses out. Until they discover a way to fit physical activity into their overwrought lives, black women—who are the most overweight and have the highest death rates from heart disease—will remain the least fit (and least healthy) of all races and genders in America.[1]

INACTIVITY IS A MAJOR HEALTH RISK

Our sedentary lifestyles are prematurely aging us from the inside out. Lack of exercise results in a weak heart that has to work harder to beat. It also makes your bones brittle, your muscles weak, your blood vessels stiff, and your midsection spread. It is impossible to be healthy without getting regular physical activity.

The consequences of our inactivity are serious. First, and most obviously, obesity and type 2 diabetes are directly linked to not burning enough calories through exercise. But excess body fat is only the tip of the iceberg when it comes to considering the health conditions either created or made worse through a lack of exercise.

Physical inactivity is to blame for our high rates of heart disease, and the reason is simple. The heart is a muscle, and like any other muscle, it becomes weak if it is not exercised. If you've ever had your arm in a cast for any period of time, you know what I'm talking about. While casted, your arm muscles cannot move. After the cast is removed, the muscles on that arm are smaller and weaker than those on your uncasted arm. In the same way, lack of regular exercise causes your heart to become weaker and pump less efficiently. Over time, a weak heart that cannot pump blood throughout the body leads to heart failure.

Physical inactivity can also be blamed for the high prevalence of high blood pressure in our community. Healthy blood vessels expand and contract with the normal changes in blood volume that occur throughout the day. Research has shown that without regular exercise, our blood vessels become stiff and inflexible. Large volumes of blood flowing through stiff blood vessels result in high blood pressure. Persistent high blood pressure is a leading cause of stroke and kidney failure, two diseases that disproportionately affect African Americans.

WHY ARE BLACK WOMEN INACTIVE?

With such obvious health benefits that require only minimal effort, why are black women the most physically inactive? The answer is that physical activity requires an investment of the most precious commodity of our day . . . time!

Before I explain, let me offer a few qualifications. Not all black women are inactive. Moreover, among those who are inactive, some black women have health problems that limit their ability to be physically active without a doctor's guidance. Furthermore, I am not implying that black women don't value our health. We do. Like most women, we make the majority of health decisions for our families. And most of us have a basic understanding of the link between physical activity and good health. But at the end of the day, many black women feel that there is simply not enough time to attend to their multiple priorities *and* find time to exercise.

There are three important trade-offs that black women must consider in order to make room for exercise. The first trade-off is caretaking. The second is hair care. And the third is body image. Before you brush these off as foolish, read on. Given the African American culture—our values, beliefs, and priorities—these are important and legitimate concerns.

Taking Care of Business

When considering the fact that black women are sedentary, many black women I know would beg to differ by saying, "How in the world can I be physically inactive when I'm busy from sunrise to sunset?" It's a fair question. For most of us, once our workday ends, a second full-time job begins. From running after the kids, cleaning the house, running errands, cooking dinner, and going to church meetings, we have miles to go before we sleep. At nightfall, we collapse in a heap, completely exhausted from the day's activities.

Because we never seem to get a moment's rest, many black women believe we get sufficient exercise performing our daily routines. But being busy does not necessarily equate to being physically active—it depends on what you're doing. If you work at a job that is relatively sedentary, your tiredness at the end of the day is related not to physical activity but to mental exhaustion. If the errands you run after work involve driving kids to sports practice, driving your mother to the doctor's office, and driving to church to sit in a meeting, then yes, you've been busy, but you have not been physically active enough to condition your heart and lungs. This constant state of activity may be mentally and physically draining, but it does not provide sufficient exercise to improve your health.

Crowning Glory

Another reason that working up a sweat may seem more trouble than it's worth is the negative effects of sweat on our hair. This may seem frivolous to some, but it is a real barrier to physical activity for black women. African American hair has a wide variety of textures and often tends to be dry. Sweat causes black hair to become even drier. Frequent shampooing is not the answer. In fact, some hairstylists recommend shampooing black hair no more frequently than every three days because daily shampooing strips the natural oils from African American hair, worsening dryness and causing breakage.

Furthermore, most black women do not have "wash and wear" hair. We spend a great deal of effort to maintain it. In beauty salons across the country, black women sit for hours every Saturday, sacrificing valuable time and spending considerable money to get their hair done. In fact, consumer surveys reveal that African Americans spend three times more on grooming than other consumer groups. Sweating during vigorous exercise means ruining a seventy-five-dollar "do." Some women tell me that they schedule their workouts immediately before their weekly salon appointments, but many women skip working out altogether.

Looking good is important, but feeling good and being around for family and friends is more important. And the two are not mutually exclusive. Options to care for black hair post-workout include using rinse-through conditioners, warm-water rinses, or light spray oil sheens. You may also consider getting braids, a blunt cut, wearing your hair in a natural style, or getting a weave. Consult your hairdresser for the best advice. But given what you now know about our increased risk of going to an early grave, please don't sacrifice your health for a hairstyle.

Fitness, Not Fatness

African Americans celebrate a wide range of shapes and sizes, and we don't shun women who carry a few extra pounds. Although being a bit overweight might motivate women of other cultures to make time for physical activity, this does not necessarily inspire black women to exercise. But it is important to understand that fitness is not just a matter of being skinny; it's a matter of being healthy. Lack of physical activity increases the risk of major health problems for all people, even those with normal weight. In fact, overweight people who exercise regularly have a lower risk for serious illness than thin people who don't exercise. As surprising as it may seem, the death rate for people who are thin

SELF-EVALUATION: YOUR EXERCISE NEEDS

Do you need to establish a regular exercise routine? Respond to each statement using the following scale:

5 = strongly agree   4 = agree   3 = neutral   2 = disagree   1 = strongly disagree

1. ___ I'd love to be more physically active, but I simply don't have time to exercise.
2. ___ If I have a choice between the stairs and the elevator, I choose the elevator.
3. ___ I don't exercise most days of the week.
4. ___ I have high blood pressure, diabetes, and/or heart disease.
5. ___ I drive to most of the places I need to go.

A score closer to 5 means that you're on the right track. If your score is closer to 25, keep reading to learn how to protect your health by fitting more exercise into your day.

and unfit is much higher than that for people who are overweight but fit.[2]

HOW TO SQUEEZE EXERCISE INTO A BUSY LIFE

Moderate amounts of physical activity provide tangible health benefits, but physical activity should not be viewed as "all or nothing." The most important aspect of physical activity is actually doing it—this means that it must realistically fit into an individual's life. There is no single "pre-scription" for achieving health-related physical activity goals, nor is there only one "right" way to reach them. Some people prefer the structure of an exercise regimen. I have found that attending weight-lifting and Zumba exercise classes at a gym is very effective for me. The "peer pressure" from my classmates motivates me to persevere until the end of each hour-long class. On the other hand, you may prefer to walk. My seventy-year-old mother walks four miles every day in the mall near her home. She has lost weight, has plenty of energy, and has lowered her blood pressure to a normal range. The one myth I want to dispel is that physical activity has to be structured in terms of type and length of time. It does not. In fact, if you lack the time and motivation to become physically active, lifestyle activities—actions performed as part of your daily routine—are a promising way to automatically increase physical activity levels. They allow you to use every opportunity to be active, don't require special equipment, cost nothing, and easily fit into your day.

WHAT IS LIFESTYLE ACTIVITY?

Do you get up every morning to walk the dog? Does your job involve manual labor? Are you responsible for the yard work at your home? If your answer to any of these questions is "yes," you regularly perform lifestyle activity. Here's another example. My son plays football. Three days a week, either my husband or I dash home after work, grab a quick bite to eat, help our son finish his homework, and rush him to the football field in time for 6 p.m. practice. Instead of waiting on the bleachers for practice to end, my husband and some of the parents jog around the football field. They not only watch their sons exercise but squeeze in some physical activity for themselves. No cost is involved, and they enjoy the companionship of other busy parents who are trying to find time to be active. Instead of having to schedule separate time to exercise, they have found a way to make exercise fit conveniently into their hectic schedule. That's the beauty of lifestyle activity. It can be done virtually anytime, anywhere, and it allows you painlessly to accumulate physical activity throughout your day.

LIFESTYLE ACTIVITY HAS THE SAME HEALTH BENEFITS AS TRADITIONAL EXERCISE

Taking the opportunity to add a bit more activity throughout your day is just as effective as going regularly to the gym. In fact, two studies comparing lifestyle activity with more structured exercise routines showed equal health benefits. At the end of two years, both groups had lower blood pressure, lower body fat, lower blood cholesterol, and comparable weight loss.[3]

Our hectic lifestyles make it more difficult to exercise, but not impossible. With some imagination and minimal effort, regular exercise can become a part of almost everyone's daily routine. Lifestyle activity overcomes the exercise barriers African American women face and is the best solution for every time-strapped person. Later in this chapter, you'll learn easy ways to incorporate exercise into your daily life. But if you're still asking, "What's in it for me?" check out the amazing ways exercise keeps you healthy.

BETTER THAN AN APPLE A DAY

The health benefits of regular physical activity are so numerous that you might find them hard to believe. But suspend your disbelief and consider the facts as summarized by the Centers for Disease Control and Prevention.[4] Physical activity:

- Reduces your risk of heart attack and stroke
- Lowers your blood pressure
- Reduces your risk of death from heart attack
- Reduces your risk of colon cancer
- Protects you from developing type 2 diabetes, even if you have been diagnosed with prediabetes
- Controls your weight
- Strengthens your muscles and bones, protecting you from osteoporosis and injury from falls

- Relieves depression and anxiety
- Improves your general well-being

WALK THIRTY MINUTES A DAY FIVE DAYS A WEEK FOR YOUR BEST HEALTH

Numerous studies have examined the health benefits of regular physical activity, and the most studied of all forms happens to be walking. Walking is the best all-purpose exercise for almost everyone, young or old, new to exercise or experienced, an athlete or a regular Joe, in good health or not in tip-top shape. The consensus is that walking at a moderate rate for at least two and a half hours a week prevents disease (fig. 7). What is a moderate rate?, you may ask. About three to four miles per hour. An easy way to determine if your pace is good is the following: if you're slightly out of breath but still able to maintain a conversation while walking, this means that you are exerting yourself at the optimal rate.

If you can spare a thirty-minute block of time, by all means you should begin a habit of walking as recommended. But if you don't have thirty minutes to spare, don't worry. It's just as beneficial to break up your physical activity throughout the day. You can find several suggestions in the "How to Move More" section of this chapter. While following these tips, an inexpensive pedometer, found in most sporting goods or retail stores, can help you monitor your progress by counting your steps. To achieve maximal health benefits, your goal should be ten thousand steps a day, which is equivalent to walking five miles. As a point of reference, the average American walks about three to five thousand steps a day (or roughly one and a half to two and a half miles a day).

JUST DO IT

Making the decision to become more physically active is a great first step. The next step is to decide which type of activity is best. In view of the seemingly limitless array of exercises you can do, you might feel over-

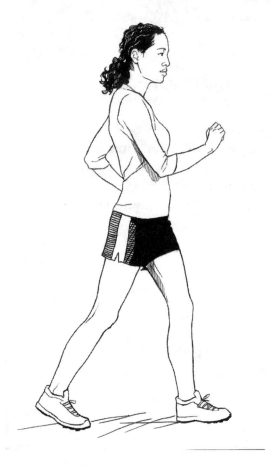

Figure 7. Walk thirty minutes a day, five days a week, for better health.

whelmed. But the most important thing to remember is this—any exercise is better than none. Stair climbing, walking, jogging, gardening, housecleaning—it doesn't matter which one. Just do it. As you begin a regular routine, it doesn't matter how long you exercise—just do it! Tonight, when you walk upstairs to your bedroom to turn in for the night, walk back down the stairs and climb them again. An extra hike up the stairs is better than none. A quiet lap around the playground is better than none. A brisk walk to the corner store is better than none. Just do it. You'll find that once you do a little, doing a little more becomes easier. The extra time in your day miraculously appears. Your lack of motivation disappears. Suddenly, five minutes of exercise becomes thirty minutes. And just as any exercise is good, more is better. The more you do, the greater the benefit you will reap.

HOW TO MOVE MORE

Luckily, exercise does not have to be a chore. There are plenty of easy ways to increase your level of physical activity while keeping to your hectic schedule.

1. Park farther from the grocery store and enjoy the walk. Instead of circling the lot in search of a parking spot close to the store, take one of the more plentiful parking spaces farther away and walk instead. Remember to wear your pedometer because every step counts.
2. Vacuum to the oldies. Load your CD player with old favorites, crank up the volume, and do your housework with pep in your step. For a 150-pound woman, vigorous vacuuming can burn 175 calories per hour. One hour of doing laundry burns 140 calories. And the housecleaning has to be done anyway. Might as well get added value from it!
3. Take a hike. At lunchtime, take a walk for fifteen or twenty minutes. And talk a coworker into going with you. Exercising with a friend makes it more likely that you'll continue to exercise, and you'll burn around 70 calories. If you keep up this habit, at the end of the year you will have lost five pounds.
4. Play like a kid. Challenge your child to a game of basketball. For a 200-pound man, a one-hour game of pick-up basketball can burn 540 calories! You'll get a great workout, and will spend quality

time with your child. Your boy or girl will appreciate the additional time he or she gets to spend with you.

5. (Window) shop till you drop. Walk briskly around the mall while you window shop. Lose weight and save money.

6. Walk, don't ride. Take the stairs instead of the elevator. And you can start small. Even if you walk one flight and ride the elevator the rest of the way to your destination, your overall well-being will ultimately improve. Once you've mastered one flight, you can try two, and then more.

7. Stop and drop. While watching your favorite TV show, drop to the floor and do ten push-ups during commercials. You'll improve your strength by building muscle. As an added benefit, your new muscle will burn fat all day, even when you're not working out.

SPECIAL CIRCUMSTANCES

You may be reluctant to exercise because you have limited mobility as a result of arthritis or other physical conditions. You may also experience discomfort because you are overweight or obese. Here are a few tips to help you get started.

1. If you have a medical condition that makes exercise difficult, your doctor can tell you what type of physical activity is right for you. If you suffer from a health problem such as heart disease or arthritis, or have mobility or joint problems, please consult your doctor before undertaking any physical activity.

2. Take it slowly. You may be motivated and excited about starting a physical activity plan. But don't go out and try to run a marathon right away. If you have been inactive for a while, allow your body to get used to an increase in activity by slowly working your way up to thirty minutes a day. If you are overweight or obese, you may only be able to get up and move your limbs for a couple of minutes a day. That's OK. Do what you can do for the first week,

and then try to add two or three minutes each week. Even two minutes of physical activity is better for your health than no activity at all.

3. Use the right equipment. If you plan to walk, the type of shoe you wear is important. Flip-flops, dress shoes, and boots are not made for walking. Get a good pair of walking shoes or sneakers to protect yourself from injury.

4. Try water aerobics or other water exercises. If you are very overweight or obese, water exercises may be more comfortable for you because they are easier on your joints.

EXERCISE MYTHS

Finally, let me dispel some common myths about exercise.

Myth #1. You must join a gym to exercise. Not necessarily. For some people joining a gym is a viable option, but you don't need a gym to exercise. Walk or jog along the sidewalks or on your treadmill. Ride your bike in your neighborhood. And while you're at it, phone a friend. Getting a friend to exercise with you will make you more likely to stick with your routine and will make exercise more enjoyable.

Myth #2. You must be in good health to exercise. Maybe. If you have a serious health condition, check with your doctor before beginning to exercise. He or she can tell you which exercises are safe for you. For many health conditions, exercise may improve your symptoms.

Myth #3. You have to buy special equipment to exercise. Nope. Something as simple as a jump rope helps you get a great aerobic workout. Cans of vegetables or jugs of water can be used as light weights. In addition, there is one type of exercise equipment that almost everyone owns . . . a pair of sneakers.

Myth #4. You have to wear special clothes to exercise. You don't need special clothes. All you need to wear in most cases is loose, comfortable clothes. An old tee shirt and a pair of loose-fitting shorts will do.

Myth #5. You have to block out a half hour of your time to exercise. It's true that at least thirty minutes of exercise every day is recommended. However, you can break up the thirty minutes into three ten-minute segments. This will help you gradually reach your thirty minutes per day goal. But even if you don't do thirty minutes a day, it's more important to do what you can do than to do nothing at all.

LET'S GET MOVING

Physical inactivity is responsible for high disease rates in the black community, and black women are the least active of all. However, our inactivity is not because we don't value our health. On the contrary, our traditional role as caretakers often leaves no time for exercise. Furthermore, legitimate hair care concerns make the average black woman think twice about working up a sweat. And our community's acceptance of overweight lessens our motivation for regular exercise.

Yet for too long our community has suffered the negative health consequences of physical inactivity—a price we can no longer afford to pay. No matter whether we are thin or fat, our health depends on our willingness to move a little bit more. African Americans no longer have to be saddled with poor health. Let's get moving.

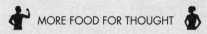

MORE FOOD FOR THOUGHT

1. Consider the modern conveniences you enjoy every day (for example, garage door opener, remote control TV, elevators). Which one(s) reduce your level of physical activity? What is one thing you can do to increase your physical activity despite these conveniences?

2. In this chapter, three barriers that prevent black women from exercising are listed (caretaking obligations, concerns about hair, and acceptance of excess weight). Do you know a black woman who is facing one or more of these barriers? (It may be you!) What can you do to help her overcome one of these barriers and become more physically active?

3. Name three conditions that physical activity prevents.

4. How much exercise is beneficial?

5. Think about your daily routine. If you're too busy to carve out thirty minutes for structured exercise, how can you make physical activity more easily fit into your busy day? Remember that even housework, sports, and lunchtime walks are excellent ways to burn calories and become physically fit. Choose something that you enjoy and you will reach your fitness goal.

CHAPTER FIVE

Detoxify Your Life: Managing the Three Ss (Stress, Sleep, and Smoking)

My church sponsors a women's retreat every year. It provides a wonderful opportunity to restore spiritual and earthly relationships in a relaxing setting. I was particularly looking forward to a recent retreat because I needed the time away from the demands of my job. I arrived at church early and unloaded my bags from the car. After checking in, I was given a goody bag and breakfast snack. Everyone was relaxed and looking forward to a great weekend. As I boarded the bus, I spotted one of my good friends and grabbed the empty seat next to her. While we were chatting, my Blackberry buzzed. *This must be an emergency,* I thought, *because my staff doesn't usually email me about routine matters when I'm on vacation.* So I read the email. My countenance immediately changed, and my girlfriend noticed right away. "What's wrong?" she asked. I waved off her question by gesturing that I needed to make a phone call. After several phone calls and emails, the issue at the job—which was not even close to being an emergency—was over, but the damage had been done to my emotional well-being. I felt tense and my mood was decidedly sour. My girlfriend looked over at me and gently said something that I wasn't in the mood to hear.

"You know," she said, "you shouldn't have answered your Blackberry."

"But they needed me!" I responded to her.

She smiled and said, "You're on vacation! If you hadn't answered your Blackberry, they would have found someone else to deal with the situation . . . and you would not be stressed out right now!"

I gave her a sheepish grin, knowing that she was absolutely right.

WHAT IS STRESS?

Stress. Everyone experiences it to one degree or another. But as common as it is, it can be a difficult concept to pin down. Go and ask ten people to define stress, and you'll likely get ten different answers, because the thing that causes stress in one person's life is inconsequential in another's. For example, one day while driving down a busy road, the traffic signal I was approaching turned yellow. Instead of gunning through the light, I decided to stop. While slowing down, I heard a horn blowing and all sorts of commotion behind me. I looked in the rearview mirror to see a middle finger being waved at me by a decidedly unhappy driver. Apparently, he wanted to blow through the yellow light, but I ruined his plans. I remained calm, but the driver behind me was furious. In this situation, the same traffic scenario that caused one driver to erupt in road rage resulted in practically no response whatsoever from me. Although our triggers are different, how each of our bodies responds to whatever causes stress in our lives is quite similar.

The stress response is your body's way of reacting to a dangerous or threatening situation. Imagine being confronted by a large beast that is eyeing you as a tasty snack. Your body's response to this danger is to prepare you to either fight the animal or run from it. (In this instance, running is probably the smarter option!) Your brain signals your adrenal glands to release cortisol, adrenaline, and other hormones to help you respond to this immediate threat. These hormones cause your heart to beat faster to supply extra blood to your arms and legs, your liver to release glucose into the bloodstream for extra energy, and your breaths to become deeper to take in extra oxygen. Some people experience almost superhuman strength as a result of their body's response to a life-threatening situation.

Marie Payton knows the power of the acute stress response. While cutting her lawn, her riding mower got away from her and trapped her four-year-old granddaughter underneath it. Marie quickly ran over and threw the mower off the child. Her body's response to the stress of seeing her grandchild in danger enabled her to do what she normally would not have the strength to do. In fact, when Marie tried to lift the mower later, she couldn't do it.[1] In our daily lives, the likelihood of being faced down by a wild animal is minimal. But the stress response allows us to fight off or escape from other emergencies requiring quick action. Once the threat has passed, your body shuts off the acute stress response, and normal operations resume.

Stress is normal: almost everyone has dealt with intermittent stress and has experienced no lasting harm from it. Stress can even be helpful in certain situations. Consider the individual who is preparing to speak before a large audience. Even the most experienced public speakers experience a certain amount of stress; this anxiety encourages them to prepare and enables them to perform well. Intermittent stress is normal and not generally harmful.

CHRONIC STRESS

For some people, however, stress is more than an occasional response to a random threat—it is a way of life. Their daily lives generate a constant stream of anxiety that never allows the stress response to shut off. For me, technology is an offender. Didn't someone promise that computers, fax machines, cell phones, email, and voice mail would make our lives easier? I have found the opposite to be true. Modern technology means that we are accessible 24/7, and these constant interruptions divert our attention from family, friends, free time, and even sleep! When we respond immediately to every email, text message, and phone call—like I did on the way to my retreat—we relinquish control of our schedules and our sanity, and we spend our days responding to the urgent rather than the important. Unhappy marriages, unending traffic jams, ungrateful kids, unreasonable supervisors, and the unrelenting pressure to make ends meet also keep stress hormones flowing and take their toll on our well-being.

Your body's stress response system does not distinguish between the stress caused by an immediate threat to your life and that caused by your Blackberry. The same stress hormones are released in every stressful situation, no matter the cause. And therein lies the problem. Chronic exposure to stress hormones makes you sick.

The Health Effects of Chronic Stress

Chronic stress triggers migraines, knots necks, clouds thinking, interrupts sleep, ignites anger, fuels anxiety, and lowers immunity. If you can't seem to shake a cold, find yourself feeling moody, or always seem to feel exhausted, you may be suffering from the effects of chronic stress.

Over the long term, persistently high levels of stress hormones raise your blood pressure and blood sugar, lower your resistance to infections, and interfere with your sleep. The stress hormone cortisol also increases the risk of serious disease by causing fat to accumulate in your abdomen. Beyond causing the all-too-familiar middle-age spread, extra abdominal fat is metabolically active and, among other things, releases immune system chemicals into your bloodstream that increase the risk of type 2 diabetes and gallbladder disease and double the risk of death from cancer, stroke, and heart disease (fig. 8).[2]

As if ill health isn't bad enough, chronic stress also contributes to premature aging—a process marked by the death of your cells. This fact should not be completely surprising because we've all seen photographs of the president of the United States at the end of his term looking markedly grayer and more worn than when he entered office. It is suspected that stress hormones may hasten cellular death by shortening telomeres, caps at the end of chromosomes. Chromosomes—the "houses" where your genetic information is found—are in every cell. Each time your cells

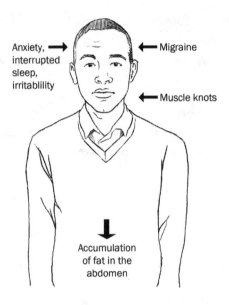

Figure 8. The health effects of chronic stress.

divide, part of the telomere "cap" wears away. When enough of that cap wears down, the cell dies.[3] This stress-induced cellular death accelerates the deterioration of the body and produces the typical signs of aging, including wrinkled skin, diminished hearing and eyesight, and weakened muscles.

The health effects of stress go far beyond the biology of stress hormones. Stress also affects our behavior. People who are chronically stressed are less motivated to take care of their health; working out and eating right seem less important. As stress builds, we stop paying attention to ourselves, and our health eventually declines from persistent neglect.

When the pressure becomes too much to bear, people who lead chronically stressful lives seek relief. It's no coincidence that Ambien (a sleep aid), Prozac (an antidepressant), and Motrin (a headache pain reliever) are top-selling medications. In addition to relying on over-the-counter and prescription meds, people suffering the misery of unrelenting stress self-medicate by overeating, smoking, drinking, and even using illicit drugs in an attempt to feel better. Whatever the choice, these coping behaviors compound the negative health effects of chronic stress.

STRESS AND AFRICAN AMERICANS

Is stress different for African Americans? Yes and no. It is true that everyone experiences stress; no race, ethnicity, or gender is exempt. It is also true that we all share common stressors. But if you are black, you can cite another important cause of stress in your life—perceived racism and discrimination.

Most African Americans have experienced being treated differently because of our race. How many black men do you know who have been pulled over because they were "driving while black"? For the uninitiated, this means being pulled over by police despite violating no laws—traffic or otherwise. Often, cops will tell them that they "fit the description" of a suspect. Many times, these men are physically and emotionally harassed by the cops simply because of their skin color.

Black women are not exempt from discriminatory treatment. On more than one occasion, I have walked through the door of an upscale shop, only to be followed around by the salesclerk as if I was planning to shoplift their merchandise!

Race-related stress on the job is another major stressor for blacks. Several years ago, I received a call from a distraught African American woman who worked in one of my programs. She was so upset that she could barely speak. She told me that her supervisor was treating her unfairly, that she was working hard but not getting the credit, and that she was denied the opportunities for promotion that were offered to the white workers in her unit. When I asked whether she had discussed this with her supervisor, she said that when she attempted to express her concerns, her supervisor threatened to "write her up" for insubordination.

I later discovered that this woman had recently returned to work after missing several days because of high blood pressure. Coincidence?

Probably not. The anxiety and stress this worker felt was real, and her body responded to it by pumping out stress hormones that raised her blood pressure.

After exploring the situation further, it was clear to me that the supervisor's actions were unreasonable and inappropriate. Although I could not definitively say that this supervisor was racist, he was clearly a poor manager. In fact, it does not matter whether this woman's supervisor was a racist or acted in a discriminatory fashion. What mattered was how the worker *perceived* the repeated incidents. This woman interpreted her supervisor's actions as discrimination, and the stress engendered by this perception manifested itself through physical illness.

Research has shown that discrimination has the same physiologic effects as marital strain, job loss, or interpersonal conflict: higher blood pressure, elevated heart rate, and lower immunity. Over time, recurrent race-related incidents can take a toll on our well-being. This type of stress has been estimated to age African Americans ten years and is a likely contributor to African Americans' high rates of chronic disease.[4]

OUR COPING STRATEGIES CAN BE HARMFUL

Although most African Americans have been subjected to discrimination, some of us are more susceptible to its adverse health effects. The difference lies in how we cope with stressful situations. Studies have shown a clear link between racial on-the-job stress and high blood pressure in African Americans. Yet not all African Americans reporting work-related racial stress showed elevations in blood pressure. The difference between the two groups was not in how they were treated (both groups felt discriminated against) but in how they *responded* to the biased treatment. The people with elevated blood pressure measurements tended to suffer in silence, whereas the people with normal blood pressure measurements were more likely to attempt to rectify the unfair treatment or at least talk about it. In other words, the most important factor was whether in response to stress they "held it in" or "let it out."[5]

It is not surprising to me that some of the workers in the study internalized their distress. Our ways of coping with adversity have been passed down from parents to their children through generations of African Americans since slavery. Stoicism and silent suffering are learned behaviors our ancestors used to overcome threats to their survival. Out of necessity, they developed these ways to cope with the inhumane treatment they endured during slavery and Jim Crow because they would be beaten if they spoke, acted, or showed any "inappropriate emotion." As Frederick Douglass explained: "[Impudence] may mean almost anything, or nothing at all, just according to the caprice of the master or overseer, at the moment. But, whatever it is, or is not, if it gets the name of 'impudence,' the party charged with it is sure of a flogging. This offense may be committed in various ways; in the tone of an answer; in answering at all; in not answering; in the expression of countenance; in the motion of the head; in the gait, manner and bearing of the slave."[6]

Today many blacks use these same coping mechanisms to deal with all kinds of stressful situations, race-related or not. Consider how we cope with the threat of ill health.

A focus group consisting of twenty-one African American cancer patients revealed that our coping style affects our pursuit of medical treatment and emotional support. The desire to be stoic in the face of adversity often keeps blacks from seeking help. One focus group participant offered this explanation, "Maybe we just tend to go within and feel like we can [cope] with it. We have had to deal with so much, you know, culturally, that maybe this is just another thing that we look at and say, 'I can handle it.'" Another focus group member said, "We tend as African Americans not to share our experiences as much. I think there's a stigma associated with seeking help. . . . For years, my mom didn't seek help because she always thought that people would see her as a weak person."[7]

Silence is often employed in an attempt to "protect" loved ones from anxiety. A focus group participant remarked, "[My father] didn't want to tell the family [about his cancer diagnosis]. He didn't want to burden us." Still another male participant said, "I have a son. . . . I don't want him going through the anxiety with me. . . . I have to hold the anxiety myself. I suffer and hold it." I personally witnessed my father, who was diagnosed with cancer in 1996 and died the same year, keep quiet about his diagnosis with everyone except his immediate family. Most of his family members learned about his diagnosis after his death. Those not familiar with our culture often erroneously interpret this silence as indifference, but like our ancestors, our silence is meant to represent our resilience in the face of adversity.

By leading us to internalize our anxiety rather than seeking outside help, our coping styles make us sick because they prevent us from seeking the medical and emotional support we need to heal. Too many times I have treated black patients who put off seeing the doctor for a suspicious lump or abnormal bleeding because deep down they were afraid of bad news. Outwardly, you would never know that anything was wrong, because they never mentioned their situation to anyone (silence) and continued with their daily lives as if nothing was wrong (stoicism). Yet this external display of strength contributes to late diagnosis and treatment of disease and is ultimately responsible for our higher death rates. African Americans must learn new and healthier ways to deal with the stress in our lives.

Our biological and behavioral responses to stress are toxic to our health. Although we can't totally eliminate stress from our lives, we can improve our health by learning how to cope with stress.

THREE STEPS TO DETOXIFY YOUR LIFE

1. Eliminate Stress

What's stressing you out? Marriage problems? Financial hardships? Work-related trouble? Stress is a part of everyday life that often can't be avoided. But we can control how we respond to stress. Holding stress in through silence or stoicism may seem to be helpful in the short term, but just like steam in a pressure cooker, as stress builds, it eventually must be released. Oftentimes, it spews out through acts of anger, sadness, vio-

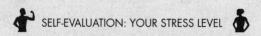

SELF-EVALUATION: YOUR STRESS LEVEL

Are you in need of healthier ways to relieve stress? Respond to each statement using the following scale:

5 = strongly   4 = agree   3 = neutral   2 = disagree   1 = strongly
   agree   disagree

1. ___ I find it hard to get more than three or four hours of sleep a night.

2. ___ I've tried to quit smoking, but every time I face a stressful situation, I light up.

3. ___ I have a great deal of stress in my life, but I just hold it in because I don't want to burden anyone with my troubles.

4. ___ I don't talk about my stress because I don't want my business in the streets.

5. ___ When strong people are stressed, they just "suck it up" and deal with it.

How are you dealing with stress? A score of 5 indicates that you're doing a great job handling stress. If your score is closer to 25, keep reading to learn how to detoxify your life.

lence, or desperation. And those are just the external consequences of unresolved stress. Internally, the constant flow of stress hormones steadily erodes your health. This is why it is imperative to learn more effective ways to handle stress. Here are several ways to cope with stressful situations.

- "Me time." Take time to recharge and rejuvenate, because you can't care for others if your tank is empty. Schedule a time for meditation or prayer, even if it's only five minutes. These stress-busters have been proven to reduce your risk of death from all causes, including heart disease and cancer, the two leading causes of death. And if you're fortunate enough to have it, by all means use your vacation time. According to a survey commissioned by Expedia.com, workers who regularly take leave report feeling more productive, rejuvenated, and connected to their families. Yet, 460 million vacation days went unused in 2008.[8] So use, don't lose, your vacation time.

- Just say no. Don't overpromise what you can't deliver, and don't feel guilty about saying no. By setting your own personal boundaries, you protect your time and your sanity. For example, don't answer emails while on vacation, and don't answer the cell phone during your family time. Furthermore, don't feel obligated to explain why you're saying no. "No" is a complete sentence.
- Ask for help. Asking for help is not a sign of weakness. No one is perfect—we all need help. Find a friend or family member to whom you can pour your heart out. It's also OK to seek counseling from either a professional counselor or a trusted pastor. Ask for a listening ear, and then go even further by asking for help or advice in dealing with the difficult situation that has you so stressed.
- Walk. In addition to its other health benefits, regular exercise is one of the best ways to counter the effects of elevated stress hormone levels. Enough said!

2. Get a Good Night's Sleep

We need seven to nine hours of sleep a night, but most of us don't get it. Why? Because we are overloaded with responsibilities on the job, at home, and in our community, and we stretch ourselves to the limit to gain enough time to do everything we need to do. High stress hormone levels, caused by the persistent stress of our 24/7 lifestyles, is a leading cause of insomnia. You may think you can get by on just four or five hours of sleep a night, but chronic sleep deprivation will ultimately affect your ability to think clearly. Sleep deprivation will shorten your attention span and make it hard for you to focus on important tasks. At best, insomnia is responsible for creating irritable, humorless people who are no fun to be around. At worst, sleep deprivation can be deadly, especially among people driving vehicles or operating heavy machinery. An estimated one hundred thousand car crashes per year are associated with people who drive while sleepy, according to the National Highway Traffic Safety Administration.[9]

You may be surprised to hear that lack of sufficient sleep is also associated with obesity. Here's how this is thought to work: sleep deprivation has been linked to a malfunction of the hormones that control your appetite. Normally, excess body fat produces a hormone called leptin that turns off appetite. New evidence suggests that lack of sufficient sleep causes signals to become crossed, which makes body fat produce less leptin and more of the hormone ghrelin—this hormone increases appetite. The results are just as you might imagine: we don't get the "I'm full" signal, we continue to eat, and we gain weight.

People who are chronically sleep-deprived are ultimately unable to regulate their sleep normally; their lives are fueled by caffeinated "energy drinks" to help keep them awake. Predictably, their high intake of caffeine also makes it difficult for them to fall asleep, so they rely on over-the-counter or prescription sleep aids. This vicious cycle entraps insomniacs into substituting chemical dependency for a good night's sleep.

Your body needs adequate sleep to rejuvenate, cope with stress, and fight disease. Two hormones, growth hormone and melatonin, are at their peak during sleep. Growth hormone heals tissues and stimulates your immune system. Melatonin does even more to protect you from illness by inhibiting tumor growth, preventing infections, increasing the number of antibodies in your saliva, and extinguishing the damaging effects of free radicals.[10]

How to Get a Good Night's Sleep

Follow these steps to enjoy the full restorative benefits of a good night's sleep:

- Go to bed at the same time every night, even on weekends.
- Finish your last meal early (at least four hours before bedtime).

Otherwise, the process of digesting your food will interrupt your sleep.

- If you have trouble getting seven to nine hours of sleep, don't drink caffeine after noon. In addition to coffee, tea, cola, and chocolate, beware of medications that contain caffeine (for example, over-the-counter pain relievers like Excedrin, some weight-loss medications, and some cold medications).
- Avoid nicotine. Like caffeine, it is a stimulant.
- Be careful with alcohol. It may help you fall asleep but may interrupt your sleep.
- Try a glass of warm milk. It contains tryptophan, a sleep-inducing agent. Tryptophan is also found in bananas, honey, and oats.

3. Stop Smoking

Although everyone knows about the deadly effects of smoking, many African Americans still rely on smoking to relieve the stress of modern living. Smoking may provide temporary stress relief, but its long-term effects turn out to be much more harmful than the stress itself. It is the leading preventable cause of death, taking the lives of more than four hundred thousand Americans every year. About 25 percent of African Americans smoke, and more than forty-seven thousand die each year from this deadly habit, most from lung cancer but many from heart disease.

If you are a smoker, the smoke your cigarette gives off harms both you and the people around you. Does your child have a cold that just won't go away? Does your grandson take medication for asthma? Do you get frequent bouts of bronchitis? Cigarette smoke is likely to blame. It contains more than four thousand chemicals that irritate your lungs and predispose you to respiratory disease.

Is Smoking Worse for Blacks?

Although cigarette smoking is a significant health threat for everyone, it is particularly harmful for African Americans. On average black smokers take in 30 percent more nicotine per cigarette, and nicotine is broken down more slowly in African Americans. This is noteworthy because the longer nicotine lingers in your system, the more nicotine you crave and the more cigarettes you smoke. The more cigarettes you smoke, the greater your risk of smoking-related disease and death.[11]

Mentholated cigarettes, preferred by approximately 75 percent of black smokers, are a major concern because they slow the body's metabolism and clearance of nicotine.[12] Even nonsmokers are familiar with popular mentholated brands of cigarettes because they are heavily advertised in the African American community. Smoking cigarettes of any type is deadly for African Americans, but given what we now know, the targeted advertising of mentholated cigarettes in the black community is particularly outrageous.

The Benefits of Quitting

Once you've made the decision to quit smoking, you won't have to wait long to reap the health benefits. Almost immediately, your heart rate and blood pressure will drop, and the levels of carbon monoxide in your blood will also become lower. Within months, your lung function will improve, and within a few years, your risk of developing smoking-related diseases will decrease to close to the risk of someone who never smoked.

There are several ways to quit smoking. Some smokers are able to stop cold turkey. They make the decision to stop smoking, and from that point on they never pick up another cigarette. Most smokers, however, need help to quit. Fortunately, there are several options from which you can choose.

- You can purchase over-the-counter nicotine replacement medication in the form of patches, gum, or lozenges.
- Your doctor can write a prescription for nicotine nasal spray, nicotine inhalers, and medications such as Wellbutrin and Chantix.
- Counseling, usually in combination with over-the-counter or prescription meds, is another option that has helped many former smokers quit.

- Even hypnosis and acupuncture have been used successfully. Talk to your doctor to decide which methods are best for you.
- You can call the American Cancer Society's Quit Line for help and advice in quitting smoking (1–800-QUIT NOW or www .cancer.org). The Quit Line can help you devise your best plan for successful quitting and refer you to low-cost or free smoking cessation services in your area.

Whichever method you choose, please remember that it may take you more than one attempt to stop smoking. Keep trying. You can do it!

Stress, sleeplessness, and smoking are toxic for African Americans. More than an inconvenience, they can be seriously damaging, even deadly to our health. Ridding our lives of these toxins takes us one step closer to the healthier life we all want.

MORE FOOD FOR THOUGHT

1. Review this list of the top ten stressors. Which one(s) are you facing? Which one of the strategies listed above can help you deal with your stress in a healthier way?
   a. Death of a spouse
   b. Divorce
   c. Marital separation
   d. Jail term
   e. Death of a close family member
   f. Personal injury or illness
   g. Marriage
   h. Fired from job
   i. Marital reconciliation
   j. Retirement
2. Have you been dealing with a long-term stressful situation? It is sometimes hard to open up to others about your problem, but holding it in is harmful to your health. Is there anyone you trust enough to talk to about your stress (for example, a pastor, a close family member or friend, or a professional counselor)?
3. If you're having trouble losing weight, it may be related to your not getting enough sleep. Think back over the past several months. How much sleep do you get on average? Do you think you need more sleep? If so, which of the strategies will you try first?
4. Smoking kills forty-seven thousand African Americans each year, more than murder, drug and alcohol abuse, car accidents, and AIDS combined. If you need to quit smoking, which strategy will be the most helpful place for you to start?

CHAPTER SIX

Change Your World: Righting the Wrongs of Social Inequity

If there is no struggle, there is no progress. Those who profess to favor freedom and yet depreciate agitation, are men who want crops without plowing up the ground, they want rain without thunder and lightning. They want the ocean without the awful roar of its many waters. This struggle may be a moral one, or it may be a physical one, and it may be both moral and physical, but it must be a struggle. Power concedes nothing without a demand. It never did and never will.
—Frederick Douglass, August 4, 1857

In the previous chapters we have seen that being healthy ultimately boils down to cultural attitudes, values, and beliefs that influence how we eat, how often we move, how much we weigh, and how we handle stress. A broader set of environmental and social factors, however, affects our ability to make these decisions. In other words, the ability to eat right and exercise regularly is not simply a matter of motivation but is influenced by your zip code, your income, your education, and your race. Years of exclusion from equal opportunities in employment, education, and wealth accumulation have resulted in an unequal distribution of the resources each American needs to be healthy. Despite notable achievements among many African Americans, blacks overall are playing catch-up on a field that is not level. As long as the imbalance remains, disparities in health will continue.

114

Therefore, to understand fully why African Americans continue to get sick and die at higher rates than any other racial group in the nation, we must consider the different features of our society that both harm and heal. For example, although race relations are now measurably different, our country's historical legacy of race has left a lingering impact on African American health. Our unequal burden of illness is not simply a medical issue—it is also a social and legal issue, a cultural inheritance of poor health that began almost four hundred years ago. To better understand the complexity of this matter, we must first review our history in America.

OUR INAUSPICIOUS ARRIVAL IN AMERICA

In 1619 the first African slaves arrived on the shores of North America. Our ancestors' voyage began in Africa, where fellow countrymen kidnapped and herded Africans from the interior of the continent to the west coast. It has been estimated that as many as 50 percent of the twenty million captives did not survive the transit to the coast. Those who survived were imprisoned in holding caves known as "slave factories" for up to several months before being exchanged for shiploads of cloth, iron, gunpowder, and firearms brought by European slave traders. Three hundred to four hundred Africans were herded down into the belly of each slave ship, a space not built for human occupation and therefore incapable of accommodating the most basic human needs. These black men, women, and children—branded with irons, shackled together, and tightly packed head to foot—sailed for up to two and a half months surrounded by human waste and their sick and dying fellow captives. They were fed and watered once a day. This voyage was known as the Middle Passage because it was the middle leg of a three-way trip made by the slave traders: from Europe to Africa, from Africa to America (by way of the West Indies), and from America back to Europe (fig. 9).

Between 10 and 20 percent of the enslaved Africans didn't survive the long trip across the Atlantic to the Caribbean and the Americas. Starvation, disease brought on by the unsanitary conditions on the ship, or

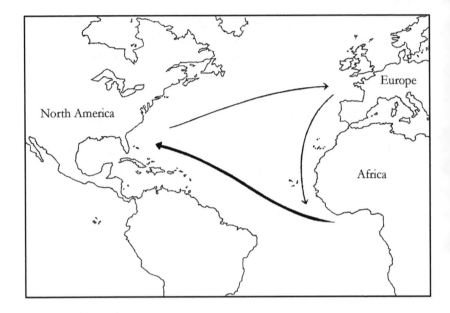

Figure 9. The Middle Passage.

suicide claimed their lives. (The fact that most of our ancestors survived the transport is a testament to our strength and resilience in the face of inhumane circumstances.)

Once they reached American soil, newly arrived African slaves were subjected to a several-month-long "breaking-in" period. They underwent the process of "deculturation," in which they were stripped of their African culture. They were forbidden to practice their native religion, speak their native tongue, or receive formal education. The stress of being torn from familiar environments and customs, along with their exposure to new diseases and climates in America, resulted in an estimated 30 to 50 percent death rate during this period.[1]

For two and a half centuries, blacks lived in servitude in the United States. During that time, black slaves were considered to be property, unworthy of the basic rights afforded other human beings. Black slaves worked from sunup to sundown. Their extreme exertion under appalling working conditions, poor nutrition, and inadequate clothing exacted a physical toll that would have brought down those of weaker constitutions.

SILENT ANGUISH

Slave families lived in silent anguish, with the constant threat of families being torn apart, babies being ripped from mothers' arms, wives being sold away from their husbands. Consider these recollections from former slaves:

> "I have seen slave mothers fall over in a dead faint when their children were sold away from them. The mothers would have to hand down their children and when they fell over in a faint men would pick the poor women up and carry them away just as if they were dogs. Those mothers loved their little children just the same as white mothers love their little babies, and some of them were never happy again and some went insane as did my old mother when her children were sold away from her."—Samuel Hall, Iredell County, North Carolina[2]

> "It was some time after this, that I married a slave belonging to Mr. Enoch Sawyer, who had been so hard a master to me. I left her at home, (that is, at his house,) one Thursday morning, when we had been married about eight months. She was well, and seemed likely to be so: we were nicely getting together our little necessaries. On the Friday, as I was at work as usual with the boats, I heard a noise behind me, on the road which ran by the side of the canal: I turned to look, and saw a gang of slaves coming. When they came up to me, one of them cried out, 'Moses, my dear!' I wondered who among them should know me, and found it was my wife. She cried out to me, 'I am gone.' I was struck with consternation. Mr. Rogerson was with them, on his horse, armed with pistols. I said to him, 'for God's sake, have you bought my wife?' He said he had; when I

asked him what she had done; he said she had done nothing, but that her master wanted money. He drew out a pistol, and said that if I went near the waggon on which she was, he would shoot me. I asked for leave to shake hands with her, which he refused, but said I might stand at a distance and talk with her. My heart was so full, that I could say very little. I asked leave to give her a dram: he told Mr. Burgess, the man who was with him, to get down and carry it to her. I gave her the little money I had in my pocket, and bid her farewell. I have never seen or heard of her from that day to this. I loved her as I loved my life."—Moses Grandy, Camden County, North Carolina[3]

When slaves became ill, they were tended to by an assortment of black root doctors, midwives, and spiritual healers. Because American diseases were foreign to these "health care providers," treatment was often inadequate. White medical providers were seldom involved in treating black slaves. The combination of heavy physical labor, poor nutrition, mental distress, and insufficient medical care gave slaves a higher death rate than whites.

A TENUOUS EMANCIPATION

In 1863, in the midst of the Civil War, President Abraham Lincoln issued the Emancipation Proclamation, an executive order that emancipated slaves in most states. Two years later, in 1865, the institution of slavery in the United States was formally abolished through the ratification of the Thirteenth Amendment to the Constitution.

Although the practice of slavery ended, African Americans did not receive equal rights under the law. They were second-class citizens, and although the law allowed them to exist in "separate but equal" status with whites in this country, there was no equality for blacks in America. The passage of Jim Crow laws, mainly in the southern states, beginning in the last quarter of the nineteenth century, established a legally endorsed system of segregation and ensured white and black separation. African Americans were unable to eat in the same restaurants, drink from the same water fountains, use the same restrooms, or receive the same medical care as whites. Threats of physical and psychological intimidation were used to keep blacks "in their place." Any African American who crossed the line might be lynched, a savage form of execution—usually by brutal beating and public hanging—with no benefit of due process. The lynch mob served as self-proclaimed judge, jury, and executioner.

"Jim Crow" was challenged in *Plessy v. Ferguson,* heard by the Supreme Court in 1896. The highest court in the land upheld the artificial "separate but equal" standard so that for nearly one hundred years, the segregation of United States citizens by race was permitted by law. The civil rights movement represented blacks' rejection of the unjust notion of segregation and second-class status. What followed were a number of landmark decisions that marked the end of legal discrimination.

In 1954, the Supreme Court's decision in *Brown v. Board of Education* desegregated the nation's public schools. In 1963 and 1964, important legal decisions made racial discrimination in hospitals illegal. These decisions were followed by the Civil Rights Act of 1964, which prohibited discrimination in all federally funded programs. In 1965, the Medicare and Medicaid programs were established. In concert, these actions attempted to end the long history of segregation and inadequate health care for blacks.

Yet the poor health of African Americans persisted. This fact was most notably documented by the 1985 *Report of the Secretary's Task Force on Black and Minority Health.* Established by the secretary of health and human services, this task force investigated the long-standing differences between minority health and white health and found "a continuing disparity in the burden of death and illness experienced by Blacks and other minority Americans as compared with our nations' population as a whole." The task force found that if minorities and whites died at equal rates, sixty thousand minority deaths would be prevented each year. They also found that six conditions were responsible for more than 80 percent (forty-eight thousand) of those deaths: cancer, heart disease and stroke, cirrhosis of the liver (from alcoholism), diabetes, homicides and accidents, and infant mortality.[4]

In the two and a half decades since these findings, African Americans have continued to get sicker and die younger than whites. Why do racial groups that share the same country and, theoretically, the same opportunities—people whose only difference is race—have dramatically different disease and death rates? One may assume that these racial differences in health reflect racial differences in biology. Is the African American race genetically predisposed to poorer health? Are we a biologically inferior race? To answer this question and better understand the issue of African American health requires first an understanding of what race is . . . and isn't.

THE HISTORY OF RACE

In the seventeenth and eighteenth centuries, Europeans ventured into foreign lands to expand their empires. During these expeditions, they encountered people who were physically and culturally different. They classified these individuals according to physical attributes and geographic location. In fact, our current racial categories are based on a system of racial classification developed in the late eighteenth century by Johann Friedrich Blumenbach, a German scientist. Blumenbach described five racial categories based on physical appearance (such as skin color, hair, and body type) and geography: Caucasian, Mongolian, Ethiopian, American, and Malay. He further described a racial pecking order that ranked Caucasians as "superior" and darker races as "inferior."[5]

An early prominent voice proclaiming blacks' racial inferiority was Thomas Jefferson, author of the Declaration of Independence. In 1781 Jefferson published his *Notes on the State of Virginia,* in which he said, "I advance it therefore as a suspicion only, that the blacks, whether originally a distinct race, or made distinct by time and circumstances, are inferior to the whites in the endowments both of body and mind." His view gained wide acceptance, and helped rationalize slavery, segregation, and discrimination against blacks.[6]

Scientific "studies" conducted before the Civil War concluded that people with dark skin, broad noses, and full lips (that is, the darker races) had weak constitutions, were genetically more susceptible to diseases like tuberculosis and pneumonia, and therefore were not fit for freedom or citizenship. Ironically, despite their frailties, they were considered to be fit for the extreme manual labor upon which this country was built. These antebellum studies "played a central role in representing blacks as inferior, inherently diseased, and . . . members of a different species."[7]

Race Is *Not* Biology

More than two hundred years have passed since Jefferson's treatise was disseminated, and contemporary scientists have discredited the notion of biologically distinct races. Genetic studies have revealed that race does not account for human genetic variation. In fact, there is more genetic variation within the African American race than between African Americans and whites. All credible scientists affirm that the African American race is not genetically inferior. Race, in fact, has no basis in biology. It is a social designation based on outward appearance, and it does not accurately reflect our genetic makeup.[8]

SOCIAL INEQUALITY CAUSES HEALTH DISPARITIES

Yet, African Americans' greater burden of illness is undeniable. Rather than being caused by our biological makeup, however, it is directly related to our ancestors' having lived in a time when individual rights, roles, and opportunities were meted out according to race. Race decided which child had the right to learn to read, which individual had the right to vote, and which family had the right to own land. Race decided which home you could buy and which neighborhood you could live in. Race decided which doctor you could see, which hospital you could enter, and which hospital door you could walk through. Generations of systematic deprivation, exclusion, and inequality have left African Americans with-out the generational wealth and educational attainment necessary for a long, healthy life. Put another way, slavery, postslavery segregation, and the artificial "separate but equal" standard resulted in segregated and in-ferior schools, jobs, housing, income, and health care for African Ameri-cans. Our poor health was, and is, directly related to our history of rela-tive economic, educational, and residential poverty.

Let me share a story that perfectly illustrates this important concept. I entered the Johns Hopkins University School of Medicine in Baltimore in the mid-1980s. During orientation of the first-year students, one of the first things we learned was the proper pronunciation of the name of the school. It was *Johns* Hopkins, not *John* Hopkins. One of the next things we learned—not during formal orientation sessions but by sheer observation—was that this prominent institution of higher learning, which trained some of the finest doctors in the world and treated some of the wealthiest and most famous patients in the world, was located in the most illogical of places. Johns Hopkins is in East Baltimore, a poor, predominantly black community with boarded-up row houses, neglected parks strewn with trash, and stark-looking public schools. The unemployment rate is high. Men congregate on street corners, and young mothers braid their children's hair on the stoops in front of their houses. This could have been the place where the phrase "concrete jun-gle" was coined, because there is certainly more concrete than grass or trees.

How incongruous it was that the most preeminent health care facil-ity rich with resources could coexist with such poverty and lack of re-sources. The irony was not lost on many of us. Most of the patients we saw were not rich, prominent, or famous. They were folks from the 'hood: lower- to middle-class African Americans struggling to make it from day to day.

I trained at Johns Hopkins for seven years—four years of medical school followed by three years of pediatrics training. During that time, I became close to many of my patients. I got to know them and their families, and they shared with me some of their deepest hopes and dreams. They were the same dreams we all share: to provide a better life for themselves and their families. Some of my patients had fairly decent jobs, but most had low-wage jobs, if they were able to find work at all. Their homes had the basic necessities but not many frills. Their communities, however, exposed them to health risks far beyond those threatened by bacteria and viruses. Regular gun violence made the streets unsafe, especially after dark. (At one time, the murder rate in Baltimore approached 365 deaths in a single year, an average of one homicide every day!) If my patients' health was not imperiled by violence, there were two other prevalent environmental threats: lead poisoning caused by exposure to chipping lead paint in poorly maintained old row houses and asthma caused by exposure to environmental toxins including cigarette smoke, dust mites, and roaches.

Many of the adults in the families had a high school education . . . or less. This low level of education affected the jobs they could get. In earlier decades, Baltimore was an industrial town, and people without college degrees could get good, stable jobs with benefits at places of employment like Bethlehem Steel. But those factories had long since shut down, leaving residents with few employment options and no health benefits. Many who were lucky enough to find seasonal work or jobs in the service industry were still unable to obtain health care coverage because their new jobs did not offer health insurance as a benefit of employment. So I typically saw these families only when their health needs were urgent, for example, if a child was in acute respiratory distress from an asthma attack. Some families were able to obtain partial Medicaid coverage—typically for the children only.

My medical education at Johns Hopkins was valuable in many ways. Besides the obvious privilege of training alongside the best medical minds in the world and the prestige of training at the top-ranked hospital in the United States, I was also made a better doctor because of what I learned from my patients. I was inspired by their ability to survive and thrive in an environment that gave them no advantages. I also learned that health was about more than just medical care; it was about one's environment, community, employment, and education.

I learned that achieving and maintaining good health are much easier in a supportive environment. I also learned that our country has room for a great deal of improvement. We live in a country where forty-six million people can't get medical treatment when they need it because they have no health insurance. We live in a country where prescription drugs are practically unaffordable for the sickest people in our communities. We live in a country where people can't be physically active because their neighborhood sidewalks are in disrepair, there are no affordable community recreation facilities, and their communities are unsafe because of the threat of violent crime. We live in a country where people can't eat right because the only affordable foods available in their neighborhoods are the fattening and salty choices found on the "value menus" of the fast-food joints on every corner, and the closest supermarket is two bus rides away.

PLACE MATTERS

A growing body of scientific literature supports what I learned in East Baltimore. To paraphrase an important program spearheaded by the Joint Center for Political and Economic Studies, "Place Matters." Poor social conditions cause poor health. The ability to achieve the most basic level of wellness is dependent on access to resources that sustain health. Inadequate social, economic, and environmental conditions are structural forces that place good health out of arm's reach for the disadvantaged. America's history of racial inequality means that more than any other group, African Americans disproportionately fall into that category.

And so, telling people simply to eat right and exercise is hollow advice for the millions of citizens who lack the resources to do so. It takes more than willpower to maintain a healthy lifestyle. Individuals are healthier in communities that are healthy.

SELF-EVALUATION: YOUR COMMUNITY'S HEALTH

Does your community provide an environment that supports good health? Respond to each statement using the following scale:

5 = strongly agree   4 = agree   3 = neutral   2 = disagree   1 = strongly disagree

1. ___ My neighborhood does not have a well-stocked supermarket. I have to do my food shopping at corner stores.
2. ___ I have plenty of fast-food restaurants in my neighborhood.
3. ___ My neighborhood's sidewalks are either in disrepair or non-existent.
4. ___ Several streetlights in my neighborhood don't work.
5. ___ I don't feel safe walking around my neighborhood after dark.

How healthy is your community? A score of 5 means that your neighborhood helps you maintain a healthy lifestyle. If your score is closer to 25, keep reading to learn how we can make our communities healthier.

TAKING CARE OF OURSELVES AND EACH OTHER

What is the most productive route out of this downward spiral of ill health in our community? To start, those of us who have the resources to do so—and that includes most of us—must take good care of our own health. But we can't stop there. We must also remember our brothers and sisters who need a helping hand. Reversing the negative trends of African American health requires that we commit to improving our communities. And everyone can make a difference, no matter how small. Here are several places to start.

1. Become politically active. Write letters to elected officials asking that they pass zoning ordinances limiting the numbers of liquor

stores and fast-food restaurants in poor neighborhoods. Also ask them to provide incentives to entice supermarkets and farmers' markets to locate in needy communities.

2. Become an active member of the PTA to ensure that schools make their tracks, playgrounds, basketball and tennis courts, and baseball fields available for safe after-hours physical activity.

3. Start a health ministry at your church or other place of worship. Offer aerobics and health education classes for members and the surrounding community.

4. Attend community association meetings. Encourage officers to invite speakers to educate residents on how to eat healthfully.

5. Organize a neighborhood watch program that works with law enforcement to make your neighborhood a safer place for children to play and adults to walk.

6. Work with local governmental agencies to ensure that they use their resources (dollars and people) to build recreational facilities in the neediest neighborhoods, provide proper upkeep to existing facilities, and work with citizens to keep communities clean.

7. Ask your doctor not only to treat you when you're sick but to show you how to stay well.

OUR UNFINISHED CIVIL RIGHTS BATTLE

The United States is now the home of black billionaires, black CEOs, black political leaders, and a growing black upper class—evidence of the hard-won victories in our fight for civil rights. The same triumphs in health have not occurred. By some measures, our health has worsened in the past half-century. Fifty years ago, blacks had a lower death rate from cancer than whites and our death rate from heart disease was comparable to that of whites. Today African American death rates from cancer and heart disease are 30 percent higher than those for whites. We cannot begin to solve our health crisis until we attend to the legacy of this country's protracted history of racial inequality. The social and economic standing of African Americans—influenced in part by this country's racial past— has contributed appreciably to the poorer health of African Americans. We must commit to changing our health for the better, and we must get involved in changing our communities for the better.

The battle has not yet been won. Too many African Americans live in poverty, are uninsured, and face racism and discrimination every day. We must battle not only against these and other injustices but also against complacency—the thought that it doesn't matter what I eat or whether I smoke (or where I live), because "I've gotta die of something." As long as we have the ability, we cannot leave as unfinished the battles that our ancestors fought. Because of their sacrifices, our lives are much better than theirs ever were. But better isn't good enough.

Yes, we must lament our current circumstances, but we must also act to change them. We are defined not by our poor health but by our faith, inner strength, and determination. This is how those in America who believed that all people should be treated equally shook off the shackles of slavery, rejected the racism of Jim Crow, leapt toward the liberation of the civil rights movement, and now embrace the electoral success of our first black president of the United States. We can change African American health for the better, one individual and community at a time.

 MORE FOOD FOR THOUGHT

1. How do healthy communities create better individual health?
2. How do we create healthy communities?
3. How does past discrimination affect overall present-day African American health?
4. Review the list of action items for creating healthier communities. Which one are you willing to start doing now? How will it help the health of your family and neighbors?

PART

III

Navigating the Health Care System
What Every African American Must Do Now

Know Your Family History

In the first two sections of this book I have described the African American health dilemma and its causes. The clear take-home message is this: as African Americans, you and I are at higher risk of getting sick. In this final section I will outline what every African American must do now to get and stay well.

As important as it is to know our general risk of disease, it's even more important to know your personal risk. That's why every African American needs to know his or her family history. Your family history is an early warning system that alerts you about certain diseases for which you may be genetically predisposed.

Some people confuse the concept of genetic predisposition with inherited diseases caused by a genetic abnormality. Sickle cell anemia is an example of an inherited disease—if you are born with two sickle cell genes, you will have sickle cell anemia. Although this purely genetic disease more commonly affects African Americans, it statistically contributes minimally to our poorer overall health status. According to the National Institutes of Health, about 70,000 Americans (this number includes mostly African Americans, but also some Hispanics) suffer from sickle cell anemia.[1] This number is dwarfed by the millions of blacks with heart disease, diabetes, cancer, stroke, high blood pressure, and obesity—conditions that are not purely genetic, but are thought to have a genetic component. Therefore, a family history of one or more of these diseases does not guarantee that you will get the disease, but only warns you that you may be predisposed toward that disease. This warning provides you an opportunity to reduce your risk of disease. For example, if two relatives in your family suffered a heart attack before the age of fifty, you have a higher risk of heart disease. You can decrease your chances of getting heart disease by getting regular checkups, monitoring your cholesterol, exercising thirty minutes a day, and maintaining a healthy weight.

A family history is easy to collect, and helpful to you, your children, your parents, and your other family members. One final point: although your spouse's family history is not relevant to your health, it's a great idea for you and your spouse to explore your family health histories together.

COLLECTING YOUR FAMILY HISTORY

Collecting a family history is relatively easy if you have a small family. If your family is large, it may seem like an impossible task. Fortunately, you don't need to talk to every single family member. Start with your parents, brothers, sisters, and children. These are your closest relatives, and are known as first-degree relatives. You and these family members are most likely to share the same genetic tendencies for certain diseases. Next, move to your second-degree relatives. These include your grandparents, aunts, uncles, nieces, and nephews.

To make the process as easy as possible, choose an event when your first-degree relatives are already together. If you're like most families, you and your relatives gather at least two or three times a year. Birthday parties, anniversary celebrations, family reunions, and holiday gatherings like Christmas, Thanksgiving, or Easter dinner provide an ideal opportunity to talk. You could even start the conversation at a Sunday dinner. To break the ice, you might consider inviting a guest speaker to discuss a health topic with your family.

Although some of your family members will have absolutely no problem discussing their health history, others may be reluctant to discuss their health. This is not unusual. As African Americans, we tend to be very private about our medical conditions, especially if they involve stigmatized matters like mental health conditions or cancer. Let your family members know ahead of time that you want to interview them, and explain why. Also explain how the information you gather can help the both of you. While some family members may feel comfortable talking to you face to face, others may prefer to answer a questionnaire, respond to an email, or talk over the phone.

What to Ask

By asking just five questions, you will learn a wealth of valuable information about your family history of disease. Here are the questions you should ask:

1. What is your date of birth?
2. What is your ethnic background? (Some family members may be a mixture of ethnicities.)
3. Have you ever had the following conditions? If yes, how old were you when you were diagnosed? (Here I list only the six conditions that are the focus of this book. But you should feel free to ask about other conditions like asthma, birth defects, alcoholism, learning problems, mental illness, and so on.)
   a. Cancer
   b. Heart disease
   c. Diabetes
   d. Obesity

e. High blood pressure

f. Stroke

The last two questions will help you gather information about deceased family members.

4. How is the deceased family member related to you (grandmother, great uncle, and so on)?

5. What were the date and cause of his or her death?

There are several ways to document your family history data. You can use a simple notebook or type "family health tree" into your Internet search engine and download a family tree online. An excellent online family health history tool is My Family Health Portrait, found at https://familyhistory.hhs.gov.

Sometimes important family health information is not readily available. For example, my father died of lung cancer in 1996. He was an only child, and both of his parents died before he did. His health information is vital in assessing my health risk because he is one of my first-degree relatives. So what are my options for learning more about his health? My mother is an excellent source of information. Because they were married for thirty-four years before he died, she can provide a good description of his health as an adult. To learn more about his childhood health, I could ask my father's first cousins, who grew up near him.

Death certificates can provide important information about the cause of death of family members, and the age of death. Some families record important health information in family Bibles. Even obituaries may include important health information.

If You're Adopted

If you're adopted and don't know your birth parents, there are resources that can help you discover important health information about your birth family. These resources can be accessed online or through the agency that arranged your adoption. Your adoptive family may also have helpful information on the health history of your birth parents.

WHAT TO DO WITH YOUR FAMILY HISTORY

Now that you've collected this information from your family, what do you do with it? Two things: store it and share it.

Store your family history somewhere safe but easily accessible. Remember to update the information at least once a year. Share the information with your family members and your children to help them protect their health. Also schedule a doctor's appointment so that you and your doctor can review your family history and assess your health risks.

You are considered to be at *high risk* of disease if one first-degree relative had early onset of disease, if you had two first-degree relatives with that disease, or if you had two second-degree relatives with that disease and one had early onset (defined as age fifty-five or younger). For example, you are at high risk if:

- Your father had a heart attack at age forty-five (one first-degree relative with early onset heart attack).
- Your mother and your sister had breast cancer (two first-degree relatives with breast cancer at any age).
- Your grandfather and your uncle had a stroke, and your uncle's stroke occurred at the age of fifty (two second-degree relatives with stroke, one with early onset).

You are at *moderate risk* of disease if one first-degree relative had a disease or if two second-degree relatives had the disease. For example, you are at moderate risk if:

- Your mother is a diabetic (one first-degree relative with diabetes).
- Your aunt and your grandfather are diabetics (two second-degree relatives with diabetes).

You are at *average risk* of disease if one second-degree relative has a disease or if no family member has a disease. For example, you are at average risk if:

- Your nephew has high blood pressure (one second-degree relative with high blood pressure).
- None of your family members has had prostate cancer.

To summarize, when analyzing your family history, you and your doctor will ask four important questions:

1. Are there any diseases that occurred at a younger age than normal (that is, before the age of fifty-five)?
2. Are there diseases that several family members had?
3. Did someone in your family have a condition that was unusual for their gender? For example, did a male family member have breast cancer?
4. Do certain combinations of diseases run in your family (such as diabetes and heart disease)?

If the answer to any of these questions is "yes," your risk for disease is higher than normal. The next step is to determine how to reduce your risk.

HOW TO REDUCE YOUR DISEASE RISK

For most diseases, family history is not enough to seal your health fate. To increase your chances of detecting a disease early or preventing it altogether, your doctor should use your family history to create your personalized disease prevention plan that recommends the type and frequency of health diagnostic and screening tests, needed treatments and changes in lifestyle, and genetic testing. For example, women are advised to get mammograms every two years starting at age fifty. However, if your family history places you at higher risk (for example, your mother and aunt were diagnosed with breast cancer in their thirties), your doctor should modify your recommended mammogram schedule so that you start at a younger age and get screened more frequently. Your doctor should also recommend that you get genetic counseling because scientific research has identified specific genes that are linked to breast cancer. You and your family members need to know whether you are carriers of these genes. In addition to being closely followed by your doctor, you will also want to eat a healthier diet, exercise regularly, maintain a healthy weight, and avoid smoking, stress, and other toxic exposures as outlined in the previous chapters.

By collecting your family history, you can identify the specific conditions that you and your family are at higher risk of getting and develop an effective plan to reduce your risk.

 MORE FOOD FOR THOUGHT

1. Based on what you already know about your family history, are there any conditions for which you might be at higher risk?

2. Is your family planning a large gathering in the next few months? Would family members be willing to spend a bit of time discussing family history and disease risk? If not, what can you do to make them feel more comfortable?

3. Do you feel comfortable discussing your family history with your doctor during your next physical exam? Based on what you now know, be sure to ask your doctor the following questions:

   a. How often should I be screened?

   b. How should I modify my health habits, such as diet and exercise?

CHAPTER EIGHT

Understand Your Health Insurance

To say that health care is expensive has to be the understatement of the year! Try going to the doctor for a routine checkup. And don't even think about getting sick or going to the emergency room. If the illness doesn't kill you, the medical bills will! Rising medical costs place a strain on working families. In fact, medical bills are a leading cause of personal bankruptcy in this country.

So how do you protect your health while protecting your pocketbook? Health insurance. It protects you from financial ruin due to a medical catastrophe, makes sure you can get the health care you need when you need it, and helps keep you healthy by allowing you to obtain preventive health services.

If you're like most Americans, your health insurance is provided through your employer. If you are poor, disabled, or over the age of sixty-five, your insurance is probably provided by a government program, namely Medicaid or Medicare.

On the other hand, forty-six million Americans have no health insurance. For this group—disproportionately populated with African Americans and other ethnic groups of color—money for health care comes out of the same family budget used to put food on the table, buy clothes for the family, and cover other necessities. When someone gets sick, working poor families without health insurance face an unfair choice that those of us with health insurance don't have to make: either get a checkup or get groceries for the family. Most uninsured families choose to cover their most immediate needs—food, clothing, and shelter—and delay seeking medical attention until a health condition becomes unbearable. A woman I met a few years ago demonstrated just how unjust this choice can be.

THE PLIGHT OF THE UNINSURED

Several years ago, I led the implementation of a public health program that provided free colon cancer screenings and treatment to people without health insurance. We advertised the program on radio spots, televised public service announcements, and printed brochures. One of our brochures landed in the hands of a woman I'll call Sandra, one of our county's one hundred thousand uninsured individuals. By the time she learned about our program, she had been suffering from abnormal bleeding and abdominal pains for some time but could not afford to get examined by a doctor. She was worried that something might be seriously wrong because two of her family members had died of colon cancer. Sandra's husband happened to see one of our brochures and showed it to her. She called our toll-free number and was immediately scheduled for an exam and a colonoscopy. Within a few days of seeing the doctor, Sandra received the news that she most feared: her tests were positive for colon cancer. But instead of being bad news, this was the best news she could have received, because within a week she was on the operating table receiving free, lifesaving surgery. Sandra's colon cancer was caught in its early stages, thanks to our program, and after surgery, her doctors declared that she was cured.

Sandra's story would not have had such a happy outcome if she had not discovered our free program. She had already fallen into the all-too-familiar pattern of not getting the health care she needed because she was uninsured. Eventually, her cancer would have progressed to the point that she could no longer bear the discomfort. By that time, however, the disease would probably have been incurable. In fact, the uninsured are more likely than people with health insurance to suffer poor health and premature death.[1]

Options for the Uninsured

It would appear that people without health insurance are doomed to suboptimal health. Granted, unlike Canada and the United Kingdom, the United States does not offer its citizens universal health coverage. But the 2010 federal health care reform legislation will expand coverage options for those who were previously unable to afford health insurance or could not qualify for health insurance because of preexisting conditions, for example (table 16). For more information on the health care reform legislation, go to www.healthcare.gov or www.aarp.org.

In addition, almost every state offers low- to no-cost health care options. Both government programs and the private health care sector provide access to checkups, health screenings, hospital and specialty care, and medications at low or no cost for people without health insurance. Here are a few resources:

1. *Health departments.* The city, county, and state health departments of most states have programs that cover primary care, specialty, screening, and treatment services for residents without health insurance. Primary care services are those that take care of your family's basic health care needs. Examples include regular checkups for children and adults, acute care for conditions such as colds or minor injuries, and screening for weight, blood pressure, vision, and hearing. Specialty care programs might provide family planning or prenatal care services. Other important screening services may include colonoscopies for individuals over the age of fifty or otherwise at risk for colon cancer and mammograms for women over forty or otherwise at risk for breast cancer. And many of the

cancer screening programs pay for treatment if needed. Some states even provide assistance in paying the partial or total cost of your prescription drugs. Check with your local or state health department for details about programs offered in your state. You can find contact information in the telephone book or online.

2. *Federally qualified health centers.* Certain parts of your state may have been designated as "medically underserved areas" by the federal government. What this means is that the federal government has determined that there are not enough doctors or health care providers in these areas to take care of the health needs of its citizens. Typically, a large number of people without health insurance reside in these areas. The federal government provides funding for clinics to be placed there, and the clinics usually charge what is called a "sliding fee" based on income. The lower your family income, the less you have to pay for health care services. If your family income is very low, you don't have to pay anything for health care. These clinics provide checkups, some screening services, and treatment. Visit the Bureau of Primary Health Care's website at http://www.bphc.hrsa.gov to find health centers in your area.

3. *Charity clinics.* In some states, private charities or religious organizations offer free clinic services to residents. The services provided by these clinics vary, and the clinic hours also vary. Your health department is probably very familiar with these clinics and can help you find a free clinic in your area. Your church and some of the larger charities in your area may also have information. If you have access to the Internet, you can go to http://covertheuninsured.org/stateguides, click on your state, and receive lots of information about free or low-cost health care resources in your area.

4. *Hospitals.* Many states have public hospitals that provide emergency hospital services for people without health insurance. In other words, these hospitals won't turn you away just because you don't have insurance. Some of these hospitals may bill you for services you receive, but almost all of them are willing to work out a payment plan. Check with your state health department for hospitals that fall into this category.

Table 16. Selected health care reform provisions

2010	2011
Health insurance companies cannot drop your insurance coverage if you get sick.	If you reach the Medicare Part D "donut hole," the cost of your brand-name prescriptions will be discounted by 50 percent. The cost of your generic prescriptions will be discounted by 7 percent.
Health insurance companies cannot place lifetime limits on your coverage.	Medicare recipients will receive free preventive health services such as annual exams, mammograms, and other screenings for cancer and diabetes.
Your adult child can remain on your health insurance policy through age 26.	
A temporary health insurance program (also known as a "high-risk pool") will be created to provide you with coverage if you have a preexisting condition.	
If you reach the Medicare Part D "donut hole" in 2010, you will get a $250 rebate to defray the costs of your prescription drugs.	
Eligibility will be expanded to allow states to cover more people under the Medicaid program.	

2014	2020
Health insurance companies will not be able to refuse to cover you because of your preexisting conditions.	The Medicare Part D "donut hole" will be completely eliminated.
If your employer doesn't offer health insurance, you will be able to purchase affordable coverage through health insurance exchanges.	

5. *State insurance administrations.* Most states have an insurance department or board that can provide you with information on low-cost health care for uninsured individuals.

IF YOU HAVE INSURANCE, USE IT WISELY

If you are fortunate enough to have health insurance, take advantage of the opportunity to see the doctor regularly, not just when you're sick. I know that's easier said than done, because over the years I've become very good at delaying doctors' appointments. But as I've gotten older, I have realized that I need to be proactive about my health not only for my sake but so I can continue to take care of my family. So I've learned to drop the excuses and make time for what's truly important. And if I can do it, you can too!

There are two general types of health insurance: fee for service and managed care. The basic differences between the two are as follows. Fee-for-service plans generally allow you to choose any doctor or hospital you want. In the past, this was the most common type of health insurance. This type is also generally more expensive than managed-care plans, which typically cost you less money but allow you less choice over the doctors you are allowed to see and the hospitals you can use. Since most Americans are covered by managed-care insurance plans, I will discuss them in more detail below.

There are three basic types of managed care: HMOs, PPOs, and POS plans. Unlike traditional fee-for-service insurance, which pays for care *after* it is delivered, managed care pays doctors and health care providers *in advance* for their services. Here is a general description of each type.

An HMO, or health maintenance organization, is a type of prepaid insurance plan that supplies medical care through a provider network—a group of doctors, nurses, other health care professionals, and hospitals that have contracted with your HMO. HMOs are the least expensive of the three types of managed-care plans. As a member of an HMO you will be assigned to a primary care doctor who will help you determine the types of health care services you need and refer you to specialists when necessary.

A PPO, or preferred provider organization, allows you more flexibility in the types of health care services you can receive. It combines features of both fee-for-service insurance and an HMO. You can use providers and hospitals both in the plan's network and out of its network. However, you will pay more for going outside the network. Referrals are not needed to receive specialty care. This type of health plan is usually more expensive than an HMO.

A point of service plan (POS) falls somewhere between an HMO and a PPO in terms of cost and flexibility. It is similar to an HMO but allows you more choice. If you belong to a POS plan, you can either be referred by your family doctor to an in-network provider (lower cost to you) or choose see an out-of-network provider without a referral (higher cost to you).

Most managed-care plans limit the medications you can use to those on their approved list, or formulary. Drugs that aren't listed on the formulary are not covered by your insurance plan. To use an unapproved medication usually means that you will have to pay its full cost.

HOW TO GET THE MOST FROM YOUR INSURANCE

Every insurance plan has rules. Rules on which doctors you can see. Rules on which services are covered and which aren't. Rules on what portion of your health care bill you're responsible for paying. Rules on advance notification before you seek emergency room care. To choose the right insurance for you and not end up paying surprise medical charges, you need to know the rules.

Rule #1: Medical Networks

Your ability to choose your doctor, hospital, or other health care provider depends on the type of health plan you join. HMOs allow the least choice, POS plans are less restrictive, and PPOs allow you the most choice.

If you have established a long-term relationship with a doctor you trust, find out whether he or she participates in your health plan by checking the plan's provider network online or calling your doctor's office. You can also request a provider network manual from your health plan. If your family doctor is not on the list of approved providers, you can still see him or her by choosing a POS or PPO health plan. Be prepared to pay a bit extra for the out-of-network provider option.

Rule #2: Covered Services

Health plans differ in the types of services they cover and in how you can access those services. Most health plans cover basic primary care but differ in the types of specialty care they cover. If you have a medical condition requiring special care, make sure your health plan covers these services. Otherwise, you may have to pay for these services yourself or you may not be allowed to access these services.

Rule #3: Your Medical Bills

Although your health plan will pay for most of your medical bill, you are responsible for paying part of it. Depending on the rules of your health plan, you may be responsible for certain payments. These are known as out-of-pocket expenses. Here are the most common:

- Deductible. This is the amount you are required to pay for health care services before your insurance will start to pay for anything. For example, if your health insurance has a thousand-dollar deductible, you must pay for the first thousand dollars of your yearly medical costs before your insurance kicks in.
- Copayment. This is the amount you must pay at every medical visit, typically between ten and twenty-five dollars per visit.
- Coinsurance. This is the percentage of the cost of your health care that you are required to pay after your deductible has been met. It usually depends on whether you received services in-network (you pay lower percentage) or outside the health plan's network

(you pay higher percentage). For example, if you have a thousand-dollar deductible and 10 percent coinsurance, after you have paid the first thousand dollars of your yearly medical costs, your coinsurance requirement means that you will pay 10 percent of the cost of every additional health care visit. So, for a five-hundred-dollar medical bill, you must pay fifty dollars.

Rule #4: Preauthorization

Some health plans require that you get permission from them before seeking certain types of care, such as emergency room care. If you don't get this permission, they may refuse to pay for the health care visit. Study the rules of your health plan so that you are aware of this requirement.

SPECIAL SITUATIONS TO CONSIDER BEFORE SELECTING A HEALTH INSURANCE PLAN

If You Leave Your Job

What if you leave the job that provided you with health insurance? Can you keep your health policy? Under a provision called COBRA (short for the Consolidated Omnibus Reconciliation Act of 1985), you can continue to be covered by your former employer's group health insurance policy for between eighteen and thirty-six months. You are responsible for paying the full cost of the group health premium during this time.

Preexisting Conditions

What if you have a chronic disease, such as kidney failure, and need health insurance? Before the health care reform act of 2010, many health plans would not cover what they call "preexisting conditions"—that is, health problems that existed before you sought to enroll in their health insurance plan. The way this usually worked is that if you had a preexisting condition, any claims to pay for services related to caring for that condition would not be covered by the health plan for a certain period of time. Health care reform means that you can no longer be discriminated against by a health insurance company if you have preexisting conditions. Temporary coverage began in 2010, and by 2014, no health plan will be able to refuse to cover you because of preexisting conditions.

MAKE SURE YOU'RE COVERED

If you are uninsured, investigate the free and low-cost resources provided earlier in this chapter to make sure you get the health care you need.

If you have health insurance, choose your health plan carefully. To review, HMOs tend to be the least expensive, PPOs tend to be the most expensive, and POS plans usually fall somewhere in between. But cost should not be your only consideration. A health plan that is low in cost may not be cost-effective in the long run if its doctors, hospitals, and other facilities are inconveniently located, causing you to miss valuable time from work and requiring you to travel long distances.

Managed-care plans should provide you with a plain-language description of all of their covered services and benefits. Most plans also have an ombudsman, a person who is available to help you understand the plan and its requirements. Your job's benefits coordinator is another important source of information. If you are having difficulty getting information from your health plan, your benefits coordinator may be able to help you. If even the benefits coordinator is having trouble, this may be a sign that you don't want to choose this plan! Try to get as much information as possible before choosing a health plan. Review all of your health insurance plan options and choose wisely.

MORE FOOD FOR THOUGHT

1. If you don't have health insurance, now is the time to explore your options, *before* you face a medical crisis. Call your local or state health department today and tell them you are uninsured. They will help you identify low-cost government or private health coverage and explain what you may be eligible for under the 2010 health care reform legislation. Each year, thousands of people across the country discover that they qualify for assistance.

2. Today, review the rules and requirements of your health plan. If the manuals make your eyes glaze over, call your plan and ask to speak to the ombudsman. Ask this person any questions you may have about your plan.

3. Go to www.healthcare.gov or www.aarp.org to learn how you can benefit from the 2010 health care reform legislation.

CHAPTER NINE

Choose the Right Doctor

I f you live in an area where you are fortunate enough to have a choice among several doctors or health care providers—and most of us do—it's important to choose wisely. Choosing the right provider takes time but is one of the most important decisions you will make. A good one knows you well and understands how to keep you healthy. In fact, when choosing a provider, you should consider the same factors that you might mull over with any other relationship.

To narrow down your choices, start with word-of-mouth recommendations from people you trust. If your friends have had a good experience with a provider, then she or he is worth considering. Another good source for referrals is your current provider, especially if you are looking for a specialist. You can also check with your local hospital. Most large hospital systems provide physician referral services.

Once you have a few names, find out whether any of the providers on your list is a participating provider with your health plan. Many health plans limit your choices to doctors who participate in their provider networks.

In order to make the best choice, consider interviewing two or three providers. These interviews will allow you to ask questions that will help you make your decision. Be aware, however, that your insurance may not pay for this visit. Before you schedule the interview, ask the provider's office whether and how much you will be charged. Also, when you call to make the appointment, ask whether the provider is accepting new patients.

PAGING DR. RIGHT

The following questions will help you choose the best doctor or other health care provider for your individual needs.

1. Are you compatible? You and your provider should get along. This makes sense, because he or she is going to know you more intimately than almost anyone else. You need to be comfortable enough to be completely honest with your provider so that he or she will have enough information to help you stay well. If your personalities clash, your provider-patient relationship won't work.

2. Is your provider compassionate? Your provider's "bedside manner" is important. Choose one who communicates with you respectfully and who seems to care about your needs. This is especially important for men. In fact, studies have shown that one of the reasons black men don't go to the doctor as often as they should is that they feel that most doctors have an uncaring attitude toward their health. As the saying goes, people don't care what you know until they know that you care.

3. Does your doctor have the proper credentials? We have all heard horror stories about people claiming to be physicians and practicing medicine or surgery on unknowing patients. How can you be sure your doctor is legitimate? At a minimum, your doctor should have a medical degree from a reputable institution and should have an active license to practice medicine in your state. You can

check your state's physician licensing board website to confirm your doctor's licensure status and see whether any complaints have been lodged against him or her. You also want to choose a physician whose medical knowledge is up to date. Many states require that doctors take continuing education classes in order to renew their license to practice medicine. A better way is to choose a doctor who is board-certified in his area of specialty. This tells you that your doctor has periodically taken and passed an exam certifying that he or she knows the current standards of patient care. For example, I am a pediatrician certified by the American Board of Pediatrics.

4. How conveniently can you access your provider? If you work and your provider does not have evening or weekend hours, you will be forced to use your leave time for medical appointments. If you don't have leave time—you may have just started a new job, for example—you're often forced to delay medical treatment in order to not risk losing your job. To avoid this dilemma, choose a provider who offers evening hours to accommodate working patients. Furthermore, location may be important to you. Some people prefer a provider with an office close to home; others prefer one close to work. If you rely on public transportation, you may want to choose a provider who is easily accessible on bus or subway routes. Finally, find out where lab tests and X-rays will be done if you need them. Some providers are able to do these tests and procedures in their office, but if you will be required to go off-site, make sure that location is easily accessible for you.

5. Who covers for your provider when he or she is away? Even doctors take time off. And wouldn't you know that the day you have a health emergency, your provider is on vacation. Who will take care of you when your doctor is away? Make sure it's someone you get along with. If you don't like the doctor who covers when your provider is away, you may want to take this into consideration when choosing a physician.

6. Other factors to consider before making your choice:
   a. Will the provider's office process your insurance claims? Some offices do this for you, while others expect you to do it for yourself. If you must submit your own insurance claims, you may have to pay for the visit up front and then be reimbursed by your insurance company. Find out in advance to avoid unpleasant surprises.
   b. Is gender important to you? For example, I have girlfriends who refuse to see a male obstetrician/gynecologist. If the provider's gender is a concern for you, check that before you decide.
   c. What about the office staff? I knew a colleague who was considered to be an excellent doctor but had several dissatisfied patients because they considered her front-office staff to be rude, inconsiderate, and uncooperative. Check out the staff while you're checking out the doctor.
   d. How long does it take to get an appointment? Let's say that you come down with the flu. Do you have to wait two weeks for an appointment? You shouldn't have to. Most physicians reserve a few slots every day for patients who need to be seen right away. If you're sick, you should be able to get an appointment within forty-eight hours.
   e. What type of provider do you need? Your primary care doctor (family doctor) should be an internist or a family practitioner. Your child's primary care doctor should be a pediatrician or family practitioner. A woman also needs an obstetrician/gynecologist. If you are a senior citizen, you may consider choosing a geriatrician, a doctor who specializes in the diseases that come with aging.
   f. Is your doctor on staff at a hospital? Try to choose a doctor who is on staff at one of the top hospitals in your area. That way, if you have to be hospitalized, you'll be comfortable with the hospital your physician uses.
   g. Does your provider understand your religious faith? Does he

or she understand your need to pray, or does he or she ridicule your beliefs? Just as a doctor who understands your culture is essential, a doctor who understands or shares your religious beliefs and how they affect your health is also important.

YOUR DECISION IS IMPORTANT

Choosing the right health care provider is important for your well-being. Sometimes, despite your best efforts, you and your provider are simply not a good match, and the best decision is to part ways.

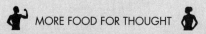 MORE FOOD FOR THOUGHT

Here are eight signs that it's time to fire your health care provider:

1. He won't explain why he's ordering tests.
2. She can't describe your medical condition in everyday language.
3. He barks out commands instead of working with you to create a realistic treatment plan.
4. You consistently experience long waits for appointments or in the waiting room.
5. She is always rushed; you never have time to ask questions or discuss your health.
6. You feel worse after your doctor's visit because you lack confidence in his decisions.
7. She doesn't take your concerns seriously.
8. He is disrespectful.

CHAPTER TEN

Schedule a Physical Exam

When was the last time you had a physical exam? If it was within the past twelve months, congratulations! You are one of the few but proud numbers of African Americans who gets a regular physical. This chapter is for those of us who haven't darkened the doorstep of our family doctor for some time.

The two most common reasons I hear for not getting a checkup are "I feel fine," and "I don't have time." Neither reason is valid. Many of the most common conditions affecting African Americans start silently. For example, high blood pressure and high cholesterol initially cause no discomfort. Early stage diabetes usually causes no pain. So feeling good is not an accurate gauge of a clean bill of health. Nor is lack of time a good excuse for avoiding the exam table. I won't go into a diatribe about how we manage to find time for every other priority in our lives and how we owe it to ourselves and our families to make the time for a physical exam and how we'll feel much better for having done so. All I will say is, Stop making excuses and schedule the exam!

Sick or not, you need to see the doctor regularly. Too many African Americans rely on trips to the emergency room or the urgent care center as a substitute for a full physical exam. If you haven't had a checkup performed by an internal medicine doctor or family physician in the last two years, it's time to schedule an appointment. In the past, yearly checkups were recommended. Today, most doctors agree that you should get a physical every one to three years.

Here are a few tips for making your appointment.

1. If possible, make the appointment for a day when you're not busy. Although your doctor will make every effort to see you on time, unanticipated emergencies can disrupt your doctor's schedule and make your wait longer than you anticipated.

2. If you know that you will be getting important tests, try to make your appointment early or midweek so you won't have to wait over the weekend for test results.

3. If there are forms that you need the doctor to complete (for example, medical forms for work or school), don't assume that the doctor will be able to fill them out during your visit. When you call to make your appointment, ask the office staff for their policy on completion of forms. Most doctors' offices ask you to allow several working days.

4. When you call to schedule your appointment, tell office staff that you will need additional time to talk to your doctor after your exam.

PREPARING FOR YOUR EXAM

No matter where I am—restaurant, business meeting, church service—someone invariably asks me about a pain, sniffle, cough, or rash. They are always apologetic after the fact, and to be honest, I don't mind answering their questions if I can. But let me suggest a better strategy. Instead of harassing some poor, unsuspecting doctor at your next cocktail party, jot down your questions in a notebook and ask them during your next physical exam. Here are some topics you might be curious about:

Your Symptoms

You may have questions about troublesome symptoms such as:

- Aches and pains
- Hair loss
- Dizziness
- Feeling tired or run down
- Unusual rashes

List all of your symptoms, no matter how trivial. Seemingly insignificant symptoms may be early signs of serious illness. For example, hair thinning or loss can be a sign of nutritional deficiency or stress. Many women with heart attacks do not have the typical chest and arm pain seen in men with heart attacks. Instead, they may experience jaw pain or nausea and vomiting. If you've noticed a change in your bowel movements, a funny-looking mole on your left arm, or a lump in your breast, don't ignore it, and don't be afraid to discuss it with your doctor.

Your Medication

You should also list questions about your medication:

- Undesirable side effects (such as diarrhea)
- Concerns that medication is not working—that is, no change in symptoms
- The need for refills
- How long you will need to continue the medication (for example, "Can I stop the medication when I feel better, or do I need to keep taking it for fourteen days?")

Make a list of all the prescription and over-the-counter medications you currently take, including vitamins and herbal supplements. Your doctor should review this list to determine whether there may be any potentially dangerous interactions. In addition, although it might be embarrassing, tell your doctor if you have tried to treat yourself by taking someone else's medication or an old antibiotic that was prescribed for you several months ago. Doctors understand that in these tough economic times, purchasing prescription medications often doesn't fit into the family's budget. But rather than resorting to taking someone else's medicine or one of your old prescriptions, consider these three options: sample medications, generic prescriptions, and prescription assistance programs. Pharmaceutical companies regularly provide free sample prescription medications to doctors' offices. Ask your doctor if he or she can give you a few samples. Second, ask for generic prescriptions, which are often just as effective as name-brand meds for less than half the cost. And third, ask your doctor to help you enroll in one of several prescription assistance programs sponsored by pharmaceutical companies or your state or local government. These programs can provide your prescription medications at low or no cost to you.

WHAT WILL HAPPEN AT THE DOCTOR'S OFFICE

If you are nervous about going to the doctor, ask your spouse, a family member, or a friend to accompany you. At your request, they will be allowed to be with you throughout the exam.

Your provider's office will probably ask you to complete several forms, so arrive early enough to fill out these forms before your exam or ask them to fax, mail, or email them to you so that you can complete them before your appointment. Some forms provide important information about your medical history. Others tell you how the office will protect the privacy of your medical information. Still others will ask for insurance information, so remember to bring your insurance card with you. Many doctor's offices will make a copy of your card for their records.

A thorough physical exam will require that you completely undress, so wear clothing that is easy to remove. Take your notebook with the list of things you want to discuss, and use it to record things you need to remember, such as the results of your exam and the doctor's instructions.

YOUR PHYSICAL EXAM

A complete physical exam consists of four basic parts:

- Medical history
- Physical exam, including screening tests
- Diagnosis
- Treatment

The first two parts, taking your medical history and performing a physical exam, allow the doctor to gather enough information to make a decision about the last two parts, your diagnosis and treatment plan.

Let's examine each part in more detail.

Medical History

The purpose of this portion of your visit is to collect information about your current illness (if any) and past medical history. The doctor will ask you to describe your current illness in detail, and will ask you about any previous illnesses, hospitalizations, and operations. He will want to know what medications you currently take, what you're allergic to, and whether any conditions like diabetes or high blood pressure run in your family. During this discussion, you should also ask the doctor questions from your notebook.

Physical Exam

The reason for your visit determines the extent of your physical exam. For example, if you are following up with your doctor for an upper respiratory illness, your exam may be limited to your head, ears, eyes, nose, throat, heart, and lungs. If you have been referred to a specialist, the examination will usually focus on the doctor's area of specialty. For example, a dermatologist will focus the examination on your skin. A complete physical, however, will be a head-to-toe examination of your body.

Don't be afraid to ask your doctor to explain your physical exam, including what he or she is doing, seeing, or feeling. Ask the doctor whether there were any problems with your exam, and record these problems in your notebook.

Screening Tests

Your doctor should order certain tests to check for diseases common to African Americans. Read the descriptions below and make sure you receive these tests at every appropriate opportunity:

1. Height and weight. Your height and weight should be measured at every visit. These numbers are used to calculate your body mass index, or BMI (see chapter 2).
2. Blood pressure. One out of every three African Americans has high blood pressure. Your doctor should check your blood pressure at least once a year. If you have high blood pressure, it should be checked at every visit.
3. Various blood and urine tests for cholesterol, sugar, and kidney function should be done every one to three years, starting at age twenty. These tests are used to predict your risk for heart disease, stroke, and diabetes.
4. HIV test. Although African Americans make up only 13 percent of this country's population, we represent half of all new HIV/ AIDS cases in the United States. Black women are being diagnosed with AIDS at higher rates than any other group in this country; the rate of AIDS diagnosis for black women is twenty-two times that for white women. It is imperative that we all know our HIV status. The Centers for Disease Control now recommends that everyone be tested for HIV. If you don't know your HIV status, ask your doctor to test you during your next visit. Testing is quick and confidential.
5. Mammogram. Black women are diagnosed with breast cancer less often than white women but are more likely to die from breast cancer once diagnosed. Younger black women are also more likely to be diagnosed with breast cancer than white women of the same

age. Current guidelines recommend that you get a mammogram every other year starting at age fifty, but because of the increased risk of being diagnosed with premenopausal breast cancer, black women should talk with their doctors about starting screening at a younger age and more often. Earlier and more frequent screening should definitely occur if you have a family history of breast cancer.

6. PSA test. Because African American men are at higher risk for prostate cancer, the American Cancer Society recommends that you talk to your doctor about drawing blood for prostate specific antigen (PSA) starting at age forty-five. Your doctor may also perform a digital rectal exam. An elevated PSA level doesn't necessarily mean that you have prostate cancer. Depending on the level, the results of your physical exam, and other factors, including your family history, your doctor will determine whether you need additional testing. ·

Diagnosis

Once the information has been gathered, your doctor will make a diagnosis. It's not unusual to have one or more diagnoses. Although it is vital that you know what you've been diagnosed with, you would be surprised by the number of people who have no idea what their diagnosis is. That's why it is best to write down the name of each diagnosis in your notebook and make sure you understand them completely before you leave the doctor's office. Ask the doctor how your diagnosis will affect your life, including your job and family responsibilities. Your doctor may also have brochures that explain your diagnosis in more detail.

Treatment

After a diagnosis is made, you and your doctor will discuss treatment options. They may include one or more medications, changes in diet and exercise, or referral to a specialist. Although doctors are experts in the diagnosis and treatment of disease, the days of "doctor knows best" are over. Any smart doctor knows that the best treatment plan is the one his or her patient will follow; achieving this requires collaboration between patient and doctor. You may be surprised to learn that there is no one single treatment for a particular condition. Your doctor usually makes a choice among several options. Therefore, if you are uncomfortable with the recommended treatment, tell the doctor that you prefer to look at other options. In addition, many treatment decisions do not need to be agreed upon immediately. Ask the doctor if you have time to think about the recommendations and discuss them with your family before making a decision.

TWELVE QUESTIONS YOU MUST ASK
AT EVERY DOCTOR'S VISIT

Getting and staying well begins with effective communication and informed decision-making about your health. You can take control of your health by scheduling regular checkups, understanding your health conditions, and working in partnership with your doctor to make healthy lifestyle choices. As a start, remember to ask these twelve questions to keep track of your health:

1. What are my weight, height, and blood pressure? Are they normal? These measurements should be performed at every doctor's visit, and you should keep track of them. Write them in your notebook along with the date of the exam.
2. Were there any problems with my physical exam?
3. What are my medical problems? What do they mean? Are they serious?
4. What are my chances for getting better?
5. What am I being treated with? How long do I have to be treated? Are there any side effects? Make sure you write down the names of the medications your doctor prescribes.
6. Is surgery or other procedure my only option? What other treat-

ment can I have instead? How many of these procedures do you perform every year? Procedures include surgery, colonoscopies, biopsies, removal of lesions, and so forth.

7. How will the results of my tests help my problem, and when will you notify me of the results? Always be sure to get the results of every test your provider orders. If you have not heard from your provider's office after two weeks, call and request your test results.

8. When do I need to return for a follow-up exam?

9. Do I need to see a specialist?

10. Does stress trigger my condition?

11. If I stop smoking, eat better, and increase my physical activity, will my condition improve? How can you help me? Your provider should discuss any lifestyle changes that might improve your condition and should provide ongoing counseling to help you through the process.

12. There are still aspects of my health that I don't understand. Would you explain them again? Can you write down your instructions for me?

MORE FOOD FOR THOUGHT

1. If you haven't gotten a checkup in a while, you might be nervous. Prepare for your next doctor's visit by using one, two, or all three of the following strategies to help calm your fears:

   a. Increase your knowledge about your health by reading books like this one. The more you understand your health, the less afraid you will be.

   b. Write down a list of questions for the doctor to help you remember what you want to ask.

   c. Ask a family member or friend to go to the doctor with you. And remember to repay the favor by being there for your loved ones when they need you.

2. More important than properly diagnosing and treating disease is preventing it. Review the list of screening tests. Are you up to date on all of them? Write down the ones you need to get and remind your doctor during your next exam.

Epilogue

In most respects, we black Americans today live lives that are quite different from when our ancestors first arrived in this country almost four hundred years ago. We have progressed from slaves to sharecroppers to landowners, from hired help to hiring managers, from laborers to leaders. Our march toward equality has been remarkable, our movement measurable. But our work is incomplete because of one obstinate disparity: the poor health of African Americans.

In this book I have explored how individual, cultural, and social factors conspire to create our predicament. Ultimately, good health is a result of life-sustaining decisions about what we consume and how we take care of our bodies. Without doubt, African American culture influences our health choices. By offering health advice in the context of the cultural beliefs and values that influence our health behavior, I have sought in *Reclaiming Our Health* to empower African Americans to create better health in our own lives, homes, and communities.

But closing the health gap doesn't stop with individual responsibility. More than knowing what to do to be healthy, we must have the resources needed to make the right decisions. Long-standing social differences between the races have affected our ability to make the best health choices. The facts are undeniable: people who are poor, unemployed, and less educated are sicker. These differences in income, employment, and education—vestiges of our country's history of race-based social inequality—affect the ability to afford nutritious foods (unhealthy fast food is often the cheapest), to engage in affordable physical activity (walking in many of our neighborhoods is dangerous), and to afford regular medical care (many low-wage jobs do not offer health insurance).

This book is far from the last word on African American health. Rather, it is a first step in the right direction. No longer can we afford to be passive participants in our health. If you're serious about reclaiming *your* health, it's time to aggressively take care of yourself and your community. Go back through these pages, retake the self-assessments, and follow the steps. Share this information with others. Help your community-based organizations fight for equity in education and employment.

Let's leave a legacy of better health for ourselves, our children, and their children—starting now!

You may have specific health and wellness questions that were not addressed in the body of this book. If so, this section is for you. Misinformation can only slow our progress toward improving African American health. Below are some of the questions I'm most frequently asked, along with their answers.

Nutrition

1. I work the night shift. How can I eat a healthy diet?

Shift workers often report disrupted eating habits and poorer diets. In general, food options are more limited during the night shift, with poorer quality of available meals and greater reliance on energy-dense vending-machine foods like candy, cookies, chips, soft drinks, and coffee. These foods tend to be high in fat, salt, sugar, and calories, and although they may give you a quick energy boost when tiredness sets in, the processed carbohydrates and caffeine found in these heavy foods can disrupt sleep during the day. Night-shift workers are also more likely to report digestive problems, including constipation and gastritis. Eating smaller, more frequent meals (for example, a sandwich, a small salad, and fruit) can help digestion. Furthermore, meals with balance of protein, carbohydrates, and a bit of fat (such as a turkey sandwich with lettuce and tomato) can help you remain alert overnight. Choose water or noncaffeinated beverages instead of loading up on the coffee or cola.

2. Are artificial sweeteners good for you? Is aspartame dangerous? Does saccharin cause cancer?

Artificial sweeteners add sweetness to foods without adding extra calories. Sugar has 4 calories per gram; most artificial sweeteners have zero calories per gram. (As a point of reference, there are 4.2 grams of sugar in a teaspoon, so a teaspoon of sugar has about 16.8 calories.) Several artificial sweeteners have been approved as safe for use by the Food and Drug Administration. Here's a breakdown of the most common sweeteners:

- Saccharin (Sweet'N Low): four hundred times sweeter than sugar. Studies in the 1970s linked saccharin to bladder cancer in lab rats. The link was never confirmed as a threat in humans, so saccharin was removed from the National Institutes of Health's list of cancer-causing agents in the early 1990s. It is currently considered safe.

- Aspartame (Nutra-Sweet, Equal): two hundred times sweeter than sugar. Aspartame should not be used by individuals with a condition called phenylketonuria (PKU). Some people develop headaches after consuming aspartame; otherwise it is considered safe.
- Sucralose (Splenda): six hundred times sweeter than sugar. Although Splenda is marketed as "made from sugar," this is technically not correct because sucralose is made by changing sugar's chemical makeup. Sucralose is considered safe.

Artificial sweeteners do not affect blood sugar, but people with diabetes should know that some foods containing artificial sweeteners—so-called "sugar-free" foods—can raise blood sugar because of other carbohydrates in the food (for example, sugar-free yogurt). In general, artificial sweeteners are relatively safe when used in moderation. But you don't want to build your entire diet around artificial sweeteners. Variety is essential to giving your body the proper balance of nutrients it needs to function, and although artificial sweeteners are calorie-free, they are also nutrient-free.

3. What is the DASH diet and how does it help my high blood pressure?
DASH stands for "Dietary Approaches to Stop Hypertension." This diet reduces your sodium intake and is filled with foods rich in nutrients that lower blood pressure (like calcium, magnesium, and potassium). It is scientifically proven to reduce your blood pressure by several points in just two weeks. Over the long term it will reduce your blood pressure even more. This healthy diet, which contains lots of fruits, vegetables, low-fat dairy products, and whole grains, may also offer protections against cancer, diabetes, heart disease, and stroke. Here is a sample day's menu from the National Institutes of Health:

Breakfast
- 3/4 cup bran flakes cereal
- 1 medium banana
- 1 cup low-fat milk
- 1 slice whole wheat bread

- 1 tsp soft (tub) margarine
- 1 cup orange juice

Lunch

- 3/4 cup chicken salad (remove salt from recipe)
- 2 slices whole wheat bread
- 1 tbsp Dijon mustard
  - Salad
  - 1/2 cup fresh cucumber slices
  - 1/2 cup tomato wedges
  - 1 tbsp sunflower seeds
  - 1 tsp low calorie Italian dressing
- 1/2 cup fruit cocktail, packed in juice

Dinner

- 3 oz beef, eye of round
  - 2 tbsp fat-free beef gravy
- 1 cup green beans sautéed with 1/2 tsp canola oil
- 1 small baked potato:
  - 1 tbsp fat-free sour cream
  - 1 tbsp grated natural cheddar cheese, reduced fat
  - 1 tbsp chopped scallions
- 1 small whole wheat roll
  - 1 tsp soft (tub) margarine
- 1 small apple
- 1 cup low-fat milk

Snacks

- 1/3 cup almonds, unsalted
- 1/4 cup raisins
- 1/2 cup fruit yogurt, fat-free, no sugar added

4. Aren't low-fat foods healthy?

Be careful with low-fat foods. Not all low-fat foods and snacks are low in calories. Many low-fat foods are high in calories because they add sugar to replace the flavor lost from reducing the fat content. So check the calorie counts.

5. Which is better for your heart . . . margarine or butter?

It depends. In my opinion, using a small amount of butter is better than using stick margarine. Here's why. Butter is high in saturated fat (raises "bad" LDL cholesterol, which increases risk of atherosclerosis), but the stick form of margarine contains trans fats, which are worse for your heart than saturated fat (because they not only raise "bad" LDL cholesterol but also lower "good" HDL cholesterol). The tub form of margarine, however, is the healthiest choice because it usually contains no trans fats. Furthermore, some brands contain plant sterols that block the absorption of cholesterol from the intestine. Many of these brands clearly indicate their plant sterol content on the label.

6. Is pork bad for you?

People seem to hold strong opinions about pork. Some believe that it is the worst food and should never be eaten. Others refuse to eat pork based on their religious or cultural beliefs. Still others, including me, have a more moderate view of pork. Although it is true that undercooked pork poses a threat to human health because it can carry parasites known as Trichinella, advances in the breeding and feeding of pork have dramatically reduced the prevalence of trichinosis in humans since the 1950s. Pork can be a great source of lean protein, B vitamins, and other essential nutrients, including iron. Chops or loin and tenderloin cuts are the best choices. To reduce the risk of disease from pork, be sure to cook it thoroughly. The Centers for Disease Control recommend cooking pork to an internal temperature of 170 degrees. Be careful about eating processed pork products, especially those cured with nitrites and salt, because of the effects on blood pressure and the increased cancer risks from foods containing nitrites. Bottom line, eating pork is a personal choice. If you do choose to eat it, do so safely.

7. How can I cook traditional foods healthier?

- Biscuits: Use vegetable oil instead of lard or butter and skim milk or 1 percent buttermilk instead of regular milk.
- Macaroni and cheese: Use low-fat cheese and 1 percent or skim milk.
- Greens—Use skin-free smoked turkey or low-fat broth instead of ham hocks. Chill chicken broth in the refrigerator. Once the fat becomes solid, skim it off before using the broth to cook greens or other vegetables.
- Gravies and sauces: Skim the fat off pan drippings. For cream or white

sauces, use skim milk and soft tub or liquid margarine. Cut the calories and fat in gravy in half by using chicken or giblet broth in place of turkey drippings. You can also cut calories and fat in dressing by cooking the mixture in a container separate from the turkey so the dressing doesn't soak up extra fat.

- Dressings and stuffing: Add broth or skimmed fat drippings instead of lard or butter. Use herbs and spices for added flavor.
- Cakes, cookies, quick breads, and pancakes: Use egg whites or egg substitute instead of whole eggs. Two egg whites can be substituted in many recipes for one whole egg. If the recipe calls for oil, replace some of it with applesauce.

8. How do I make sense of food labels?

Follow these simple steps to make reading nutrition labels—and choosing healthier foods—easier:

a. First, pay attention to the serving size, then ask yourself, "How many servings am I eating?" The nutritional information is based on a single serving size. If you eat two servings, you'll need to double the numbers.

b. Next, look at the number of calories per serving. Multiply this number by the number of servings that you're eating. The FDA considers a food with 40 calories per serving a low-calorie food. A food with 100 calories per serving has a moderate number of calories. And a food with 400 or more calories per serving is considered to be a high-calorie food. Eating too many calories per day is linked to overweight and obesity. And remember, adult females need between 1,600 and 2,400 calories per day and adult males need between 2,000 and 3,000 calories per day.

c. Now, move down to the nutrients section:

- The first few nutrients—total fat, cholesterol, and sodium—are the ones that Americans tend to get too much of. These are the nutrients you want to limit. The total fat section is broken down into saturated fats and trans fats. You want to keep these to a minimum in your diet because they are linked to heart disease, high blood pressure, and cancer. The percent daily value tells you how close this food gets you to the *upper limit* of these nutrients for the day.

- Next, look at the amounts of vitamins, minerals, and fiber. Most Americans don't get enough of these nutrients, so pay special attention to this section. The percent daily value tells you how close this food gets you to the *minimum amount* you need for the day.

- Here's how to understand percent daily value: For all nutrients, 5 percent daily value or less is low, and 20 percent daily value or more is high. If you want to eat a diet low in sodium to reduce your risk of high blood pressure, and the nutrition label tells you that one serving contains 22 percent daily value of sodium, you probably want to choose a different food because this food is high (more than 20 percent) in sodium. On the other hand, if you want to eat foods rich in iron, and the nutrition label tells you that one serving contains 5 percent daily value of iron, you may want to choose a different food because this food is low (5 percent or less) in iron.

- You will find that some nutrients, mainly protein, sugars, and trans fats, do not have a percent daily value. A percent daily value is not required for proteins because most people get sufficient protein in their diets. The only exception to this rule is if the food claims to be high in protein. For sugars, no daily reference value has been established. To keep track of the sugar in your diet, compare the labels of similar foods (for example, a couple of boxes of cereal) to determine which has the lower number of grams of sugar. For trans fats, I recommend that you completely eliminate these from your diet because they raise LDL ("bad") cholesterol and lower HDL ("good") cholesterol, thereby increasing the risk of heart disease. The best foods have 0 grams trans fats.

d. Last, look at the "ingredients" list at the bottom of the package. Ingredients are listed in order of weight (or amount) from most to least. This provides another useful way to choose healthy foods. For example, if you are trying to limit sugar in your diet, choose a food that does *not* have an added sugar as one of the first few ingredients. Alternate names for sugars include corn syrup (or other types of syrup), high fructose corn syrup, fruit juice concentrate, sucrose, honey, maltose, and dextrose. Also, check the ingredients list for "partially hydrogenated vegetable oil," another name for trans fats. Next, make sure that any bread, cracker, or bar that claims to be whole grain does not contain "enriched" flour. Whole grains (whole wheat, whole rye, and so on) should be among the first ingredients listed. Don't be fooled by the brown coloring often added to so-called wheat bread. Check the ingredients list on the bread wrapper. The shorter the ingredients list, the better.

9. How much less fat is in chicken when you bake it instead of frying?
One medium fried chicken breast with the skin has 430 calories and 17 grams of fat. If you bake the chicken breast, the counts are 380 calories and 15 grams of fat. If you bake the chicken breast and don't eat the skin, you consume only 280 calories and 6 grams of fat. One last tip: white meat is lower in calories and saturated fat than dark meat, especially when the skin is removed.

Physical Activity

1. How much exercise do I need to do to lower my blood pressure?
Regular aerobic exercise makes your heart pump more efficiently. Because it is stronger, it pumps blood through your arteries at a lower pressure. To reap the blood pressure-lowering benefits, you need to exercise thirty minutes a day for five to seven days a week.

2. I don't like to exercise. What can I do?
You are not alone! I used to hate to exercise, too. What helped me was to try different forms of exercise. I tried jogging and running on the treadmill and hated them both. I tried power walking around the neighborhood but quickly got bored. Then a friend suggested that I try taking classes in the gym. Although the first few sessions were very hard, I have grown to love it. Two things keep me going back: I've made a number of new friends in the gym, and I love the transformation of my body from flabby to fit. If you hate to exercise, try these tips:

- Try a different type of exercise, like yoga or spinning, or try the Wii video system.
- Incorporate exercise into activities you need to do anyway. For example, if you need to go to the store to pick up a gallon of milk, why not walk or bike to the neighborhood gas station or corner store instead? Or multitask by watching your favorite TV show or reading your favorite magazine or book while on the treadmill or stationary bike?
- Set a goal. Psych yourself into exercising in order to reach a specific goal, like running a mini-marathon or entering a bike race.

- Maybe what you really hate is going to a gym. In that case, buy a DVD and work out at home. Or make a regular date to play your favorite sport (tennis, basketball, softball).

3. Can weight lifting raise my blood pressure?

Yes, lifting weights causes a temporary increase in blood pressure. Remember to breathe; holding your breath during exertion causes a more dramatic increase in blood pressure. Overall, exercise is beneficial to your health. But if you have high blood pressure, check with your doctor about your weight-lifting regimen. Rather than telling you to discontinue weight lifting, he or she may recommend that you lift lighter weights for more reps.

Obesity

1. Why do we seem to gain weight once we get older?

As we age, we lose muscle mass and add fat. Muscle tissue is metabolically active and requires a lot more energy (the burning of a lot more calories) to sustain it. As our muscle cells decrease with aging, our metabolism also slows, and we gain weight. Therefore, if you eat the same number of calories as before, you have fewer muscle cells to burn those calories, and they end up stored as fat. And this process occurs at a younger age than you might think. It is estimated that we lose about a half pound of muscle mass each year starting in our thirties. Exercise helps muscles grow larger and stronger and actually helps combat the diminution of muscle mass that comes along with older age.

2. Can an overweight person still be healthy?

Yes. It is possible that you can eat right and exercise regularly and still have a body mass index that falls in the "overweight" range, especially if you have increased your muscle mass through exercise. Remember, the BMI (body mass index) is an imperfect measure of body fat. Furthermore, skinny is not synonymous with healthy. In fact, thin people who have poor diets and exercise routines are likely to be less healthy than larger people who take care of themselves.

High Blood Pressure

1. Does caffeine raise blood pressure?

Caffeine can raise blood pressure, although not everyone is sensitive to its effects. Talk to your doctor about it; he or she may recommend that you reduce the amount of caffeine in your diet (that is, drink fewer cups of coffee or caffeinated soft drinks).

2. If I feel dizzy or have a headache, does that mean that my blood pressure is elevated?

Headaches and dizziness can be indicators that your blood pressure is elevated. But these symptoms can also occur in people without high blood pressure. On the other hand, the absence of dizziness and headaches does *not* mean that your blood pressure is normal. More often than not, high blood pressure has no symptoms whatsoever. Check your blood pressure at every doctor's visit. If you have been diagnosed with high blood pressure, check it more often as directed by your doctor.

3. Are finger and wrist blood pressure machines accurate?

These types of machines are not considered to be as accurate as the machines that measure blood pressure around the arm.

4. Is sea salt healthier than table salt?

Although sea salt is often marketed as healthier than table salt, by weight they contain about the same number of milligrams of sodium. Sea salt tastes different (some say better) than table salt because it is processed differently. Also, sea salt may contain less iodine than table salt. Iodine is an essential mineral for thyroid health that prevents goiter (an enlarged thyroid). Other dietary sources of iodine include seafood, strawberries, egg yolks, milk, and milk products.

5. Does drinking alcohol affect blood pressure? What about stress?

Yes, both drinking alcohol and experiencing stress or anxiety can raise blood pressure.

6. How does salt increase blood pressure?

When you eat too much salt, which contains sodium, your body holds extra water to "wash" the salt from your body. In some people, this may cause blood pressure to rise.

7. What are hidden sources of salt (sodium) in foods?

- Processed foods such as lunch meats, sausage, bacon, and ham
- Canned soups, bouillon, dried soup mixes
- Canned vegetables
- Condiments (ketchup, soy sauce, salad dressings)

- Frozen and boxed mixes for potatoes, rice, and pasta
- Snack foods (pretzels, popcorn, peanuts, chips)
- Carry-out pizza, Chinese food, Mexican food
- Natural and processed cheeses

Diabetes

1. Does eating too much sugar give you diabetes?
No.

2. How does exercise lower my blood sugar?
If you have type 2 diabetes, exercise can lower your blood sugar by improving your body's use of insulin. Excess abdominal fat causes your body to become resistant to the effects of insulin. By burning body fat through exercise, insulin sensitivity is improved. In general, after exercise your muscles become more sensitive to insulin and absorb more sugar from the blood.

3. Can diet plans like Nutrisystem help me control my diabetes?
Yes. You've probably seen the television commercials advertising Nutrisystem D for people with diabetes. Diet plans like these can be helpful as part of a type 2 diabetes control plan for a couple of reasons. First, they tightly control your caloric intake, so they help people with type 2 diabetes lose weight. Second, many of the meals are low on the glycemic index, meaning that they are less likely to cause spikes in blood sugar. One downside of these plans is the expense—the meals can cost three hundred dollars per month on average. Of course, after you've completed the plan, you will have to maintain healthier eating habits on your own.

Cancer

1. Is it true that once air hits cancer (during cancer surgery), the cancer will spread?
No, but many people believe that it does. A 2003 study in the *Annals of Internal Medicine* revealed that 37 percent of people surveyed believed this myth. Sixty-one percent of those who believed it were African American. This finding does not surprise me, because I grew up hearing this myth. It is important for African Americans to know that surgery happens to be a very effective treatment for many cancers. In some instances, it allows the best available chance for survival. Delaying surgery can shorten your life and increase the

risk of cancer spreading throughout your body. Talk to your doctor about any concerns you may have about surgery.

Heart Disease

1. Does soy lower cholesterol?

A 1995 report in the *New England Journal of Medicine* concluded that substituting soy for some of the saturated fat in your diet allows you to reduce your LDL ("bad") cholesterol while maintaining a healthy level of protein in your diet (table 17). The Food and Drug Administration recommends eating 25 grams of soy protein per day to improve your heart health. (However, because of its estrogenlike properties, soy probably should not be used in patients with hormone-sensitive cancer such as breast, uterine, and ovarian cancer. Check with your doctor.)

2. Are heart attacks more common in the morning? Why?

Yes. In fact, it is common knowledge among doctors that the morning hours are the prime time for heart attack and stroke. A 2004 study explained why this is so. The volume of blood flowing through your blood vessels at any given time is variable—sometimes higher and other times lower. To accommodate these normal fluctuations in blood flow and maintain a normal blood pressure, your blood vessels expand and contract. This study found that blood vessels are stiffer (less flexible) in the early morning hours. In addition, levels of adrenaline—a hormone that causes a quicker heart rate and a higher blood flow—are naturally higher during the early morning hours, usually between 6 and 9 a.m. This combination of increased blood flow through stiff blood vessels places a strain on the heart and circulatory system and increases the likelihood of an early morning heart attack. Call 911 if you experience heart attack symptoms, especially if they awaken you in the early morning.

3. How is heart disease associated with Alzheimer's disease?

According to several scientific studies, including a 2004 study published in the journal *Lancet,* Alzheimer's disease is linked to atherosclerosis in mechanisms that are not fully understood. Furthermore, research highlighted by the Alzheimer's Association reveals that African Americans suffer from Alzheimer's disease, a brain disorder that destroys brain cells and causes problems with memory and brain function in older adults, at a higher rate than whites.

Table 17. Forms of soy protein

Soy protein	What is it?	How is it commonly eaten?	Protein per serving	How to use it
Tofu	Made from cooked pureed soybeans	Stir-fries; smoothies; dips; cheese substitute	4 oz firm tofu contains 13 g soy protein	Use in stews and stir-fries; takes on the flavor of whatever it's cooked in
Soy milk	Milk substitute (can be used by lactose-intolerant individuals)	Plain or flavored varieties (vanilla, chocolate, coffee, etc.)	8-oz glass contains 10 g soy protein	Add to baked goods and desserts; use in smoothies
Soy flour	Made from roasted soybeans ground into a fine powder	Found in cereals, pancake mixes, frozen desserts; also used as egg substitute		Use to thicken sauces or gravies
Textured soy protein	Made from dehydrated soy flour	Used as a meat substitute		
Tempeh	Made from whole cooked soybeans	Used as a meat substitute	1/2 cup contains 19.5 g soy protein	
Miso	Fermented soybean paste	Used as a seasoning and in soup stock		

Alternative Therapies

1. How effective is colon cleansing?

The perceived need for colon cleansing is based on the theory that undigested foods build up in the colon and release toxins that circulate throughout the body, poisoning it and causing fatigue, weight gain, constipation, low energy, and headaches. It is true that our Western diet does not contain adequate fiber and other foods that sweep the colon clean and keep the digestive system active. Popular mechanisms for colon cleansing include colonic irrigation (washing out the colon with volumes of fluid) and laxative use. These forms of colon cleansing carry certain serious risks, including dehydration, infection, perforation of the colon, and serious electrolyte imbalances. Rather than assume the risks of these methods, you should keep your colon clean naturally by eating plenty of foods high in fiber, drinking plenty of water, and exercising regularly.

2. Is noni juice effective in fighting disease? What about acai berry products?

Noni juice comes from the noni plant, a tropical evergreen tree found in the Pacific Islands, the Caribbean, and South America, among other locations. It has been touted as an effective treatment for cancer, high cholesterol, arthritis, high blood pressure, HIV, diabetes, and many other health conditions, but more research is needed to determine the validity of these statements. Because there is no current scientific evidence that noni juice can cure, treat, or prevent disease, the Food and Drug Administration has warned several companies to stop making these claims. The juice is high in potassium, which may cause problems for people with kidney disease and those taking high blood pressure medication. Other long-term health effects are unknown. Acai berries are the fruit of the acai palm tree, native to South America. Like other fruits, they are rich in antioxidants. Although research supports eating a diet rich in antioxidants to reduce the risk of heart disease, cancer, and other conditions, studies on acai berry products are limited. As with noni juice, health claims that acai berries are an effective treatment for health conditions including arthritis, obesity, cancer, and high cholesterol have not been proven. We have much more to learn about these alternative treatments. Until we do, it is unwise for you to rely on these treatments as a substitute for conventional medical care.

FREQUENTLY ASKED QUESTIONS

3. How effective are energy drinks?

Most energy drinks consist of some combination of caffeine, sugar, and other ingredients like ginseng, taurine, and carnitine. They claim not only to boost energy but also to improve mental and physical performance and protect against disease. Few studies have been performed to support or refute these claims. Although some energy drinks are sugar-free and low in caffeine, many of these drinks contain significant amounts of sugar (20 to 30 grams, or five to seven teaspoons, per eight ounces) and caffeine (80 mg per eight ounces, or roughly the same amount as in a regular cup of coffee). Check labels carefully, and limit your intake to avoid inadvertently adding inches to your waistline or becoming addicted to the caffeine in the drinks.

180

GLOSSARY

Aerobic exercise. A type of exercise that maximizes the amount of oxygen in your blood by causing you to breathe more deeply and your heart to beat faster. "Aerobic" means "with oxygen"; this type of exercise helps you maintain a healthy weight, eases stress, and makes you more fit. Examples include walking, jogging, Zumba, swimming, and basketball.

Alzheimer's disease. A condition in which brain cells die, resulting in loss of memory and mental abilities in older adults. Other symptoms include confusion, forgetfulness, change in personality, altered sleep patterns, inability to follow directions, and problems with speech.

Antioxidants. Substances that protect your body from damage caused by free radicals, harmful molecules produced during an energy-generating process called oxidation. Free radical damage is associated with cancer, heart disease, and diabetes. Here's another way to think about this process. When you slice an apple, it turns brown because of oxidation. But if you dip that sliced apple in orange juice (which contains vitamin C, an antioxidant), it remains white. Antioxidants are found in fruits, vegetables, fish, nuts, dark chocolate, green tea, coffee, red wine, and pomegranate juice. These foods contain the antioxidants selenium, lutein, lycopene, beta carotene, and vitamins A, C, and E.

Artery. A blood vessel that carries oxygenated blood from the heart to the rest of the body.

Atherosclerosis. A disease of the blood vessels in which plaque accumulates, narrows vessels, and restricts blood flow. Symptoms depend on the part of the body to which blood flow is restricted:

- Inadequate blood flow to brain = stroke
- Inadequate blood flow to heart = heart attack
- Inadequate blood flow to legs = peripheral artery disease, or claudication
- Atherosclerosis is also associated with Alzheimer's disease

Body mass index (BMI). A measure of body fat based on height and weight (see tables 8 and 9).

Calorie. A unit of energy provided by the food that you eat and drink. The energy from calories provides the fuel your body needs.

Cancer. A condition in which cells in a part of the body grow out of control and cause the loss of normal body function. Cancer is the second leading cause of death in the United States.

Carbohydrates. An essential nutrient found in foods such as breads, grains, pasta, rice, fruits, and vegetables. Carbohydrates have four calories per gram.

Cholesterol. A waxy, fatlike substance that naturally occurs in the body to help it function properly. Eating fatty foods can result in too much cholesterol in the blood, a risk factor for atherosclerosis.

Chromosomes. Long, threadlike pieces of DNA holding multiple genes. Each human cell has forty-six chromosomes, twenty-three from mom and twenty-three from dad. Two of the forty-six chromosomes are sex chromosomes (x and y) that determine whether offspring will be male (xy) or female (xx).

Diabetes. A disease characterized by abnormally high levels of glucose (sugar) in the blood. It occurs when the body fails to process sugar correctly.

Fasting blood sugar. The level of sugar present in your blood drawn a minimum of eight hours after your last meal. A value of 126 mg/dl or greater on two separate occasions seals the diagnosis of diabetes. (A normal fasting blood sugar is between 70 and 100 mg/dl.)

Fat. An essential nutrient found in foods such as butter, cream, oils, nuts, avocados, and oily fish like salmon and herring. At nine calories per gram, fats have twice as many calories per gram as carbohydrates or proteins.

Free radicals. Toxic by-products produced during cell metabolism that cause the cell damage associated with heart disease, cancer, and diabetes.

Genes. Basic units of heredity made up of DNA. Genes are passed from parents to their children and determine traits like personality, intelligence, and physical appearance.

Glucose. A type of sugar the body uses for energy.

HDL (high density lipoprotein). "Good" cholesterol that protects arteries from atherosclerosis by clearing out excess cholesterol. HDL blood level should be 60 mg/dl or more. High HDL levels are linked to a low risk of atherosclerosis.

Health disparities. Differences in the quality of health and health care across racial groups.

Heart attack. A condition in which the supply of blood and oxygen to an area of heart muscle is blocked, resulting in a decrease in the pumping function of the heart. If not treated quickly, the damaged area of heart muscle dies. Also known as myocardial infarction.

Heart disease. A variety of different diseases affecting the heart, including heart attack, heart valve disease, and congenital heart defects. Heart disease is the leading cause of death in the United States.

Heredity. The biological process whereby genetic traits are passed from parents to their offspring.

Hyperpigmentation. A condition in which patches of skin become darker than the surrounding skin. Often occurs in African Americans after scarring from acne, skin trauma, or sun exposure.

Hypertension (high blood pressure). A condition in which the force of blood against artery walls remains too high. High blood pressure is known as the silent killer because it has no initial symptoms. It can lead to heart failure, kidney failure, stroke, and other serious conditions.

Inflammation. Your immune system's natural defense against injury or irritation. Chronic inflammation may play a role in the development of conditions like cancer, diabetes, heart disease, and Alzheimer's disease.

Insulin resistance. A condition in which insulin becomes less effective in lowering blood sugar, characterized by the body's decreased ability to respond to the effects of insulin.

LDL (low density lipoprotein). "Bad" cholesterol that blocks arteries and increases the risk of atherosclerosis. LDL blood level should be 100 mg/dl or less.

Metabolic syndrome. A cluster of symptoms (high blood pressure, abdominal obesity, insulin resistance, high blood sugar, high blood cholesterol) that occur together and increase your risk of heart attack, diabetes, and stroke. Having three or more of these symptoms means you have metabolic syndrome.

Metabolism. The process whereby your body gets the energy it needs from food.

Monounsaturated fat. A healthy fat found in olives, peanut and canola oils, nuts, and avocados that lowers LDL (bad) cholesterol and reduces the risk of heart disease.

Nutrients. Chemicals that your body needs to live and grow. The six essential nutrients are carbohydrates, fats, protein, minerals, vitamins, and water. Nutrients come from a wide variety of foods, and the more varied your diet, the more likely you are to obtain all the nutrients you need.

Obesity. An excess of body fat that increases your risk of disease.

Physical activity. Any movement of the body that requires energy expenditure. Physical activity is critical for your overall health.

Plaque. A sticky material made up of fat, cholesterol, and other substances that accumulates inside the walls of arteries and reduces blood flow.

Polyunsaturated fat. A healthy fat found in fish (for example, omega-3 fatty acids). Polyunsaturated fat helps lower cholesterol levels.

Prediabetes. A condition characterized by blood sugar levels that are higher than they should be but not high enough to be diabetes. It means the cells in your body are becoming insulin resistant. Also known as "borderline diabetes," this condition means that you are at a high risk of developing diabetes. Prediabetes is defined as a fasting blood glucose level between 100 and 125 mg/dl.

Preexisting condition. A medical condition that existed before you obtained health insurance. Before the health care reform act of 2010, these conditions affected health care coverage because insurance companies either refused to cover people with preexisting conditions, imposed a waiting period before coverage began, or charged higher premiums and out-of-pocket expenses. By 2014, insurance companies will not be allowed to refuse coverage for people with preexisting conditions. Until that provision takes effect, the government's Pre-existing Condition Insurance Plan (PCIP) will make it easier for individuals with preexisting conditions to get health care coverage. For more information, go to www.healthcare.gov.

Prehypertension. An elevated blood pressure that if left untreated can become high blood pressure. Prehypertension is a blood pressure between 120/80 and 139/89.

Protein. An essential nutrient found in foods such as meat, dairy products, nuts, beans, and soy. Protein has four calories per gram.

Race. A categorization of humans into groups on the basis of physical traits. Race is not based on biology. There is no one gene or trait that distinguishes the members of one "race" from the members of another "race." There are more genetic differences within a race than between races. Race was historically used to justify social inequalities (for example, the isolation of Native Americans, the treatment of African Americans as inferior).

Saturated fat. Fat found primarily in animal sources. An excessive intake of saturated fat raises cholesterol levels and increases the risk for heart disease and stroke.

Sickle cell anemia. An inherited form of anemia that affects individuals primarily of African heritage. The disorder is characterized by crescent (sickle)-shaped blood cells that can get stuck in blood vessels and block blood flow, causing anemia, pain (sickle cell crisis), and organ damage. Sickle cell anemia is a genetic disorder; a person born with two sickle cell genes has sickle cell disease; a person born with one gene has sickle cell trait, a condition with no symptoms. Other common problems associated with sickle anemia include frequent infections, stroke, and acute chest syndrome (pneumonia-like symptoms, including shortness of breath, chest pain, and fever).

Sleep apnea. A sleep disorder associated with obesity in which breathing repeatedly starts and stops. Results in loud snoring, difficulty staying asleep, and daytime sleepiness.

Stress. The body's normal psychological and physical reaction that protects you against perceived threats. The "fight or flight" reaction.

Stroke. A condition that occurs when the blood supply to a part of the brain is disrupted, causing brain cells to die. Stroke is the third leading cause of death in the United States, and there are two main types, ischemic and hemorrhagic. Ischemic stroke, the most common type, occurs when a blood clot blocks blood flow to a part of the brain. Transient ischemic attacks (TIAs) or "mini strokes" occur when blood flow to the brain is briefly interrupted. Hemorrhagic stroke occurs when a blood vessel breaks, causing bleeding in the brain.

Trans fat. A synthetic fat made by adding hydrogen to liquid vegetable oils to make them more solid. This fat, also known as partially hydrogenated oil, is bad for your health because it raises bad cholesterol (LDL) and lowers good cholesterol (HDL). It is found in a variety of fast foods, frozen foods, stick margarine, and commercial pastries.

Triglycerides. Fatty substances in the blood. Elevated levels are often associated with obesity and poorly controlled diabetes. Some studies have found that people with high triglyceride levels are at increased risk for heart disease and stroke.

Unsaturated fat. See "Monounsaturated fat" and "Polyunsaturated fat."

Vein. A blood vessel that transports blood from the various regions of the body to the heart.

N O T E S

Chapter One AN AMERICAN INJUSTICE

1. American Heart Association, "Heart Facts 2007: All Americans, African Americans" (Dallas: American Heart Association, 2007), http://www.american heart.org/downloadable/heart/1176927558476AllAmAfAm%20HeartFacts07_ lores.pdf; National Institutes of Health, National Heart, Lung and Blood Institute, *Morbidity and Mortality: 2007 Chartbook on Cardiovascular, Lung, and Blood Diseases,* http://www.nhlbi.nih.gov/resources/docs/07-chtbk.pdf; US Department of Health and Human Services, Office of Minority Health, "Eliminate Disparities in Cardiovascular Disease," http://cdc.gov/omhd/AMH/factsheeets/cardio .htm; American Heart Association, *Heart Disease and Stroke Statistics—2008 Update,* http://www.americanheart.org/downloadable/heart/1200078608862HS_Stats %202008.final.pdf; US Department of Health and Human Services, Centers for Disease Control, "Diabetes Successes and Opportunities for Population-Based Prevention and Control: At a Glance, 2009," http://www.cdc.gov/nccdphp/publi cations/aag/ddt.htm; US Department of Health and Human Services, Office of Minority Health, "Cancer and African Americans," http://www.omhrc.gov/templates/ content.aspx?ID=2826; US Department of Health and Human Services, Centers for Disease Control and Prevention, Office of Minority Health and Health Disparities, "Eliminate Disparities in Cancer Screening and Management," http:// www.cdc.gov/omhd/AMH/factsheets/cancer.htm; Pfizer, *Racial Differences in Cancer: A Comparison of Black and White Adults in the United States* (2005), http:// media.pfizer.com/files/products/Racial_Differences_in_Cancer.pdf; US Department of Health and Human Services, Centers for Disease Control and Prevention, Diabetes Surveillance System, "Age-Adjusted Incidence of End-Stage Renal Disease Related to Diabetes Mellitus per 100,000 Diabetic Population, by Race/Ethnicity and Sex, United States, 1980–2006," http://www.cdc.gov/diabetes/statistics/ esrd/fig5; US Department of Health and Human Services, Centers for Disease Control and Prevention, Diabetes Surveillance System, "Age-Adjusted Hospital Discharge Rates for Nontraumatic Lower Extremity Amputation per 1,000 Diabetic Population, by Race, United States, 1980–2003," http://www.cdc.gov/diabetes/ statistics/lea/diabetes_complications/fig6.htm); A. M. Miniño et al., "Deaths: Final Data for 2004," *National Vital Statistics Reports* 55, no. 19 (2007), http://www .cdc.gov/nchs/data/nvsr/nvsr55/nvsr55_19.pdf; US Department of Health and

Human Services, Centers for Disease Control and Prevention, National Center for Chronic Disease Prevention and Health Promotion, *Preventing Chronic Disease by Activating Grassroots Change, 2009,* http://www.cdc.gov/nccdphp/publications/AAG/pdf/healthy_communities.pdf; US Department of Health and Human Services, Centers for Disease Control and Prevention, National Center for Health Statistics, *Health, United States, 2007,* "Table 29: Age-Adjusted Death Rates for Selected Causes of Death, by Sex, Race, and Hispanic Origin: United States, Selected Years, 1950–2004," http://www.cdc.gov/nchs/data/hus/hus07.pdf.

2. D. U. Himmelstein et al., "Medical Bankruptcy in the United States, 2007: Results of a National Study," *American Journal of Medicine* 122 (2009): 741–746.

3. US Department of Health and Human Services, Centers for Disease Control and Prevention, "Overweight and Obesity," http://www.cdc.gov/nccdphp/dnpa/obesity/faq.htm#costs; US Department of Health and Human Services, Centers for Disease Control and Prevention, "Heart Disease Facts and Statistics," http://www.cdc.gov/heartdisease/facts.htm; "Cancer: Basic Facts," in American Cancer Society, *Cancer Facts and Figures, 2005* (Atlanta: American Cancer Society, 2005); American Stroke Association, "Impact of Stroke," http://www.strokeassociation.org/presenter.jhtml?identifier=1033; Tim Dall et al., "Economic Costs of Diabetes in the US in 2007," *Diabetes Care* 31 (2008): 1–20; "About Hypertension: Prevalence, Costs, and Control," http://www.avapro-avalide.com/about_hypertension.aspx, originally published in American Heart Association, *Heart Disease and Stroke Statistics* (Atlanta: American Heart Association, 2007).

4. David Satcher et al., "What If We Were Equal? A Comparison of the Black-White Mortality Gap in 1960 and 2000," *Health Affairs* 24 (2005): 459–464.

5. M. M. Heckler, *Report of the Secretary's Task Force on Black and Minority Health* (Washington, DC: US Government Printing Office, 1985); Brian D. Smedley, Adrienne Y. Stith, and Alan R. Nelson, eds., *Unequal Treatment: Confronting Racial and Ethnic Disparities in Health Care* (Washington, DC: National Academies Press, 2003).

6. Harvard School of Public Health, Robert Wood Johnson Foundation, and ICR/International Communications Research, *Americans' Views of Disparities in Health Care,* http://www.rwjf.org/files/research/Disparities_Survey_Report.pdf; Anouk Amzel and Chandak Ghosh, "National Newspaper Coverage of Minority Health Disparities," *Journal of the National Medical Association* 99 (2007): 1120–1125.

7. US Census Bureau, "The Face of Our Population," http://factfinder.census.gov/jsp/saff/SAFFInfo.jsp?_pageId=tp9_race_ethnicity.

8. G. Howard et al., "Cigarette Smoking and Progression of Atherosclerosis:

The Atherosclerosis Risk in Communities (ARIC) Study," *Journal of the American Medical Association* 279 (1998): 119–124.

9. K. W. Lee et al., "Cocoa Has More Phenolic Phytochemicals and a Higher Antioxidant Capacity Than Teas and Red Wine," *Journal of Agricultural and Food Chemistry* 51 (2003): 7292–7295.

10. P. M. Ridker et al., "Comparison of C-Reactive Protein and Low-Density Lipoprotein Cholesterol Levels in the Prediction of First Cardiovascular Events," *New England Journal of Medicine* 347 (2002): 1557–1565.

11. C. L. Rock et al., "Reproductive Steroid Hormones and Recurrence-Free Survival in Women with a History of Breast Cancer," *Cancer Epidemiology, Biomarkers, and Prevention* 17 (2008): 614–620.

12. E. Cho et al., "Red Meat Intake and Risk of Breast Cancer among Premenopausal Women," *Archives of Internal Medicine* 166 (2006): 2253–2259.

13. L. A. Brinton et al., "Recent Trends in Breast Cancer among Younger Women in the United States," *Journal of the National Cancer Institute* 100 (2008): 1643–1648.

14. National Diabetes Education Program, "The Diabetes Epidemic among African Americans," http://ndep.nih.gov/media/FS_AfricanAm.pdf.

15. L. V. Svetkey et al., "Heritability of Salt Sensitivity in Black Americans," *Hypertension* 28 (1996): 854–858.

Chapter Two LOSE WEIGHT AND WIN

1. S. Kumanyika, "Obesity in Minority Populations: An Epidemiologic Assessment," *Obesity Research* 2 (1994): 166–182; K. Flynn and M. Fitzgibbon, "Body Images and Obesity Risk among Black Females: A Review of the Literature," *Annals of Behavioral Medicine* 20 (1998): 13–24.

2. N. Baturka, P. P. Hornsby, and J. B. Schorling, "Clinical Implications of Body Image among Rural African American Women," *Journal of General Internal Medicine* 15 (2000): 235–241.

3. M. Chandalia et al., "Metabolic Complications of Obesity: Inflated or Inflamed?" *Journal of Diabetes and Its Complications* 21 (2007): 128–136.

4. Chandalia et al., "Metabolic Complications of Obesity."

5. D. A. Dawson, "Ethnic Differences in Female Overweight: Data from the 1985 National Health Interview Survey," *American Journal of Public Health* 78 (1988): 1326–1329.

6. J. F. Hollis et al., "Weight Loss during the Intensive Intervention Phase of the Weight-Loss Maintenance Trial," *American Journal of Preventive Medicine* 35 (2008): 118–126.

Chapter Three FROM SOUL FOOD TO FOOD FOR THE SOUL

1. J. M. McGinnis and W. H. Foege, "Actual Causes of Death in the United States," *Journal of the American Medical Association* 270 (1993): 2207–2212.

2. US Department of Agriculture, Center for Nutrition Policy and Promotion, "The Healthy Eating Index, 1999–2000," http://www.cnpp.usda.gov/publications/hei/hei99-00report.pdf.

3. *The Encyclopedia of African-American History, 1619–1895: From the Colonial Period to the Age of Frederick Douglass,* ed. Paul Finkelman, 3 vols. (New York: Oxford University Press, 2006).

4. J. H. O'Keefe, N. M. Gheewala, and J. O. O'Keefe, "Dietary Strategies for Improving Post-Prandial Glucose, Lipids, Inflammation, and Cardiovascular Health," *Journal of the American College of Cardiology* 51 (2008): 249–255.

5. "Healthy Eating Index, 1999–2000"; B. M. Popkin, A. M. Siega-Riz, and P. S. Haines, "A Comparison of Dietary Trends among Racial and Socioeconomic Groups in the United States," *New England Journal of Medicine* 337 (1997): 1846–1848.

6. K. J. Joshipura et al., "Fruit and Vegetable Intake in Relation to Risk of Ischemic Stroke," *Journal of the American Medical Association* 282 (1999): 1233–1239.

7. H. C. Hung et al., "Fruit and Vegetable Intake and Risk of Major Chronic Disease," *Journal of the National Cancer Institute* 96 (2004): 1577–1584; M. Xue et al., "Activation of NF-E2-related Factor-2 Reverses Biochemical Dysfunction of Endothelial Cells Induced by Hyperglycemia Linked to Vascular Disease," *Diabetes* 57 (2008): 2809–2817.

8. Harvard School of Public Health, "Fiber—What Should You Eat?" http://www.hsph.harvard.edu/nutritionsource/what-should-you-eat/fiber/.

9. "Healthy Eating Index, 1999–2000."

10. US Department of Health and Human Services, US Department of Agriculture, *Dietary Guidelines for Americans* (2005), http://www.health.gov/dietary guidelines/dga2005/document/html/appendixB.htm.

11. HealthAssist.net, "High Blood Pressure Causes, Symptoms, Risk Factors," http://www.healthassist.net/conditions/high-blood-pressure.shtml.

Chapter Four MAKE THE RIGHT MOVES

1. US Department of Health and Human Services, Centers for Disease Control and Prevention, National Center for Chronic Disease Prevention and Health Promotion, *Physical Activity and Health: A Report of the Surgeon General* (1996), http://www.cdc.gov/NCCDPHP/sgr/sgr/htm; J. P. Seale, M. Davis-Smith, and I.

Okosun, "Ethnic and Gender Differences in Lifestyle Risk Factors in a Bi-Ethnic Primary Care Sample: Prevalence and Clinical Implications," *Ethnicity and Disease* 16 (2006): 460–467.

2. Seale, Davis-Smith, and Okosun, "Ethnic and Gender Differences," 460.

3. A. L. Dunn et al., "Comparison of Lifestyle and Structured Interventions to Increase Physical Activity and Cardiorespiratory Fitness: A Randomized Trial," *Journal of the American Medical Association* 281 (1999): 327–334; R. E. Andersen et al., "Effects of Lifestyle Activity vs. Structured Aerobic Exercise in Obese Women: A Randomized Trial," *Journal of the American Medical Association* 281 (1999): 335–340.

4. US Department of Health and Human Services, *Physical Activity and Health.*

Chapter Five DETOXIFY YOUR LIFE

1. HowStuffWorks, "How Can Adrenaline Help You Lift a 3,500 Pound Car?" http://health.howstuffworks.com/adrenaline-strength.htm.

2. T. Pischon et al., "General and Abdominal Adiposity and Risk of Death in Europe," *New England Journal of Medicine* 359 (2008): 2105–2120.

3. E. S. Epel et al., "Accelerated Telomere Shortening in Response to Life Stress," *Proceedings of the National Academy of Sciences* 101 (2004): 17312–17315.

4. A. T. Geronimus et al., "'Weathering' and Age Patterns of Allostatic Load Scores among Blacks and Whites in the United States," *American Journal of Public Health* 96 (2006): 826–833.

5. R. Din-Dzietham et al., "Perceived Stress Following Race-Based Discrimination at Work Is Associated with Hypertension in African Americans: The Metro Atlanta Heart Disease Study, 1999–2001," *Social Science and Medicine* 58 (2004): 449–461; N. Krieger and S. Sidney, "Racial Discrimination and Blood Pressure: The CARDIA Study of Young Black and White Adults," *American Journal of Public Health* 86 (1996): 1370–1378.

6. Frederick Douglass, *My Bondage and My Freedom* (New York: Miller, Orton, and Mulligan, 1855), 80.

7. A. K. Matthews et al., "Factors Influencing Medical Information Seeking among African American Cancer Patients," *Journal of Health Communication* 7 (2002): 205–219.

8. Expedia.com "Annual Expedia Survey Reveals Nearly One of Every Three American Workers Are Vacation Deprived," http://press.expedia.com/index.php?s=press_releases&item=419.

9. National Highway Traffic and Safety Administration, "Research on Drowsy Driving," http://www.nhtsa.gov/Driving+Safety/Distracted+Driving/Research+on+Drowsy+Driving.

10. Medicinenet.com, "How to Get a Good Night's Sleep," http://www.medicinenet.com/script/main/art.asp?articlekey=50595.

11. E. J. Perez-Stable et al., "Nicotine Metabolism and Intake in Black and White Smokers," *Journal of the American Medical Association* 280 (1998): 152–156; R. S. Caraballo et al., "Racial and Ethnic Differences in Serum Cotinine Levels of Cigarette Smokers," *Journal of the American Medical Association* 280 (1998): 135–139.

12. N. L. Benowitz, B. Herrera, and P. Jacob, "Mentholated Cigarette Smoking Inhibits Nicotine Metabolism," *Journal of Pharmacology and Experimental Therapeutics* 310 (2004): 1208–1215.

Chapter Six CHANGE YOUR WORLD

1. National Colloquium on African American Health, "Racism in Medicine and Health Parity for African Americans: The Slave Health Deficit" (Washington, DC: National Medical Association, 2002), http://www.nmanet.org/images/uploads/Racism%20in%20Medicine.pdf.

2. University of North Carolina Library, "Slavery in North Carolina," http://www.lib.unc.edu/stories/slavery/story/life4html.

3. University of North Carolina Library, "Slavery in North Carolina."

4. M. M. Heckler, *Report of the Secretary's Task Force on Black and Minority Health* (Washington, DC: US Government Printing Office, 1985), ix.

4. R. S. Cooper, J. S. Kaufman, and R. Ward, "Race and Genomics," *New England Journal of Medicine* 348 (2003): 1166–1170; R. M. Brewer, "Thinking Critically about Race and Genetics," *Journal of Law, Medicine, and Ethics* (2006): 513–519; Stephen Jay Gould, "The Geometer of Race," *Discover Magazine*, November 1, 1994, http://discovermagazine.com/1994/nov/thegeometerofrac441; Lundy Braun, "Race, Ethnicity, and Health: Can Genetics Explain Disparities?" *Perspectives in Biology and Medicine* 45 (2002): 159–174; E. Barnett et al., "The Social Construction of Race," in *Men and Heart Disease: An Atlas of Racial and Ethnic Disparities in Mortality* (Morgantown, WV: West Virginia University, 2001), http://www.cdc.gov/dhdsp/library/maps/cvdatlas/atlas_mens/03-section1.htm; C. J. Tashiro, "The Meaning of Race in Health Care and Research—Part 1: The Impact of History," *Pediatric Nursing* 31 (2005): 208–210.

5. Braun, "Race, Ethnicity, and Health," 159.

6. Thomas Jefferson, *Notes on the State of Virginia,* ed. Merrill D. Peterson (New York: Library of America, 1984), 270.

7. Braun, "Race, Ethnicity, and Health," 159; D. R. Williams, "Race, Socioeconomic Status, and Health: The Added Effects of Racism and Discrimination," *Annals of the New York Academy of Sciences* 896 (1999): 173–188.

8. Williams, "Race, Socioeconomic Status, and Health," 173.

Chapter Seven KNOW YOUR FAMILY HISTORY

1. Medicinenet.com, "Sickle Cell Disease," http://www.medicinenet.com/ sickle_cell/article.htm.

Chapter Eight UNDERSTAND YOUR HEALTH INSURANCE

1. Institute of Medicine, Committee on the Consequences of Uninsurance, *Coverage Matters: Insurance and Health Care* (Washington, DC: National Academies Press, 2001).

RESOURCES

GENERAL HEALTH INFORMATION

The following books provide general information on African American health:

Brock, Rovenia M., PhD. *Dr. Ro's Ten Secrets to Livin' Healthy: America's Most Renowned African American Nutritionist Shows You How to Look Great, Feel Better, and Live Longer by Eating Right.* New York: Bantam, 2003.

Collier, Andrea King, and Willarda V. Edwards, MD. *The Black Woman's Guide to Black Men's Health.* New York: Warner Wellness Books, 2007.

Gaines, Fabiola Demps, and Roneice Weaver. *The New Soul Food Cookbook for People with Diabetes.* Alexandria, VA: American Diabetes Association, 2006. *Great recipes for everyone, not just people with diabetes.*

Gaston, Marilyn Hughes, MD, and Gayle K. Porter, PsyD. *Prime Time: The African American Woman's Complete Guide to Health and Wellness.* New York: One World/Ballantine, 2003.

Gavin, James R., MD, PhD. *Dr. Gavin's Health Guide for African Americans: How to Keep Yourself and Your Children Well.* Alexandria, VA: American Diabetes Association, 2004.

Martin, Marilyn, MD, MPH. *Saving Our Last Nerve: The Black Woman's Path to Mental Health.* Munster, IN: Hilton, 2002.

Williams, Terrie M. *Black Pain: It Just Looks Like We're Not Hurting.* New York: Simon and Schuster, 2008.

The following websites provide comprehensive and reliable general health information:

American Academy of Family Physicians. www.familydoctor.org. *Comprehensive health information from a reliable source.*

Blackdoctor.org. http://blackdoctor.org. *Website with health information specifically targeted to African Americans.*

Black Healthcare.com. www.blackhealthcare.com

Everyday Choices. www.everydaychoices.org. *A collaboration of the American Diabetes Association, American Heart Association, and American Cancer Society focusing on making healthy lifestyle choices aimed at preventing diabetes, heart disease, stroke, and cancer.*

Everyday Health. www.everydayhealth.com

Health. http://minorityhealth.hhs.gov

Health day. www.healthday.com

Mayo Clinic. www.mayoclinic.com

Medical News Today. www.medicalnewstoday.com

MedicineNet. www.medicinenet.com

National Library of Medicine. http://www.nlm.nih.gov/medlineplus/african americanhealth.html. *One of the best websites for general or disease-specific information on African American health. Provides links to other websites and resources.*

New York Times. www.health.nytimes.com

Science Daily. www.sciencedaily.com

US Department of Health and Human Services Office of Minority Health. http://minorityhealth.hhs.gov

WebMD. www.webmd.com

www.health.gov. *Portal to the websites of a number of multiagency health initiatives and activities of the US Department of Health and Human Services and other federal departments and agencies.*

AFRICAN AMERICAN HEALTH STATISTICS AND DISEASE-SPECIFIC INFORMATION

American Cancer Society. *Cancer Facts and Figures for African Americans, 2009–2010.* http://www.cancer.org/acs/groups/content/@nho/documents/document/cffaa20092010pdf.pdf. *An excellent, comprehensive reference.*

American Diabetes Association. http://www.diabetes.org/living-with-diabetes/complications/african-americans-and-complications.html. *General statistics on diabetes in African Americans.*

American Heart Association. "African Americans and Cardiovascular Diseases." http://www.americanheart.org/downloadable/heart/12607254319 50FS01AF10.pdf. *A fact sheet with important statistics about heart disease and African Americans.*

Centers for Disease Control and Prevention. http://www.cdc.gov/nchs/fastats/black_health.htm. *Statistics on the overall health of African Americans.*

———. "HIV/AIDS among African Americans." http://www.cdc.gov/hiv/topics/aa/resources/factsheets/aa.htm. *Statistics on HIV/AIDS in African Americans.*

———. "National Diabetes Fact Sheet 2007." http://www.cdc.gov/diabetes/pubs/pdf/ndfs_2007.pdf. *The most current statistics available from the government's primary public health resource.*

The Henry J. Kaiser Family Foundation. "Black Americans and HIV/AIDS." http://www.kff.org/hivaids/upload/6089–07.pdf. More HIV/AIDS statistics.

National Center for Health Statistics. *Health, United States, 2009. Excellent, comprehensive listing of African American health statistics. Provides links to tables and figures containing data collected by the Centers for Disease Control and Prevention.*

National Institutes of Health, National Diabetes Education Program. "The Diabetes Epidemic among African Americans." http://ndep.nih.gov/media/FS_AfricanAm.pdf. *General statistics on diabetes in African Americans.*

National Stroke Association. http://www.stroke.org/site/PageServer?pagename=AAMER. *Statistics on stroke in African Americans.*

US Department of Health and Human Services Office of Minority Health. http://minorityhealth.hhs.gov/templates/content.aspx?lvl=3&lvlID=6&ID=301. *Statistics on heart disease, high blood pressure, and smoking in African Americans.*

———. http://minorityhealth.hhs.gov/templates/content.aspx?ID=3022. *Statistics on stroke in African Americans.*

———. http://minorityhealth.hhs.gov/templates/content.aspx?lvl=3&lvlID=537&ID=6456. *Statistics on obesity in African Americans.*

———. "HIV/AIDS and African Americans." http://minorityhealth.hhs.gov/templates/content.aspx?lvl=2&lvlID=51&ID=3019. HIV/AIDS statistics.

ALZHEIMER'S DISEASE

Alzheimer's Association. www.alz.org/africanamerican

RESOURCES

HEART DISEASE

American Heart Association. www.americanheart.org.

National Heart, Lung, and Blood Institute. www.nhlbi.nih.gov.

CANCER

American Cancer Society. www.cancer.org.

National Cancer Institute. www.cancer.gov.

HIGH BLOOD PRESSURE

Blackdoctor.org. "High Blood Pressure and African Americans." http://black
doctor.org/content.aspx?counter=126.

Centers for Disease Control and Prevention. "High Blood Pressure." http://
www.cdc.gov/bloodpressure/facts.htm.

WebMD. "High Blood Pressure in African Americans." http://www.webmd.com/
hypertension-high-blood-pressure/hypertension-in-african-americans.

STROKE

National Stroke Association. www.stroke.org.

DIABETES

American Diabetes Association. http://www.diabetes.org/in-my-community/
programs/african-american-programs. *Lists American Diabetes Associa-
tions programs specifically for African Americans.*

National Institutes of Health, National Diabetes Education Program. "More than
50 Ways to Prevent Diabetes." http://www.ndep.nih.gov/media/50Ways
_tips.pdf. *A great brochure with practical tips to not only prevent diabetes
but live a healthier lifestyle overall. The last page is a "food and activity
tracker" to help you keep tabs on your healthy eating and active lifestyle.*

IF YOU WANT TO. . . .

Eat Right

American Dietetic Association. http://www.eatright.org/Public. *User-friendly
information on food and nutrition to help you make healthy choices.*

Harvard School of Public Health. http://www.hsph.harvard.edu/nutritionsource/
index.html. *This website, maintained by the Department of Nutrition at*

the Harvard School of Public Health, provides great science-based, practi-cal information on eating right.

National Institutes of Health Office of Dietary Supplements. http://ods.od.nih
.gov/health_information/health_information.aspx. *Extensive informa-tion on dietary supplements.*

Exercise

American Academy of Family Physicians. http://familydoctor.org/online/
famdocen/home/healthy/physical/basics/015.html. *Comprehensive infor-mation on exercise for the whole family.*

National Institutes of Health, National Institute of Diabetes and Digestive
and Kidney Diseases. "Tips to Help You Get Active." http://www.win
.niddk.nih.gov/publications/tips.htm. *A downloadable booklet with help-ful tips. Especially useful if you're just starting to become physically active.*

Lose Weight

Centers for Disease Control and Prevention. "Healthy Weight." http://www
.cdc.gov/healthyweight/index.html. *Tools to help you maintain a healthy weight. Includes body mass index calculator.*

National Heart, Lung, and Blood Institute. "Controlling Your Weight." http://
www.nhlbi.nih.gov/health/public/heart/obesity/lose_wt/control.htm.
Information to help you lose weight or maintain your current weight.

WebMD. "Healthy Eating and Diet." http://www.webmd.com/diet/guide/
health-and-diet-eating-healthy. Articles and resources to help you lose
weight safely and effectively.

Quit Smoking

American Cancer Society. "Guide to Quitting Smoking." http://www.cancer
.org/Healthy/StayAwayfromTobacco/GuidetoQuittingSmoking/index.
A comprehensive resource.

Centers for Disease Control and Prevention. "How to Quit Smoking." http://
www.cdc.gov/tobacco/quit_smoking/how_to_quit/index.htm. *Provides links to several good resources to help you quit smoking.*

Smokefree.gov. http://www.smokefree.gov. *An interactive website to help you quit smoking.*

Lower Stress

American Academy of Family Physicians. "Coping with Stress." http://family
doctor.org/online/famdocen/home/common/mentalhealth/stress/167
.html. *Covers all aspects of stress and stress management.*

Collect Your Family Medical History

US Department of Health and Human Services. "My Family Health Portrait."
https://familyhistory.hhs.gov/fhh-web/home.action. A convenient online tool from the office of the surgeon general to help you collect, print,
store, and update your family medical history.

Choose a Good Doctor

American Medical Association "Doctorfinder." https://extapps.ama-assn.org/
doctorfinder/recaptcha.jsp. *Helps you locate a doctor who best meets your
medical needs. Search limited to doctors who are members of the American Medical Association.*

Consumer Reports. "Your Doctor Relationship." http://www.consumerreports
.org/health/doctors-hospitals/your-doctor-relationship/overview/
index.htm. *Comprehensive resources and information to help you choose
the best doctor, including help in checking your doctor's credentials and his
or her patients' experiences.*

Healthgrades. http://www.healthgrades.com. *Rates doctors, dentists, hospitals,
and nursing homes.*

Ratemds.com. www.ratemds.com. *Allows you to find out how your doctor's
other patients rate him or her. Also allows you to enter a rating.*

Learn More about Health Care Reform

AARP. "The New Healthcare Law: How It Impacts African Americans." http://
assets.aarp.org/www.aarp.org_/articles/health/hcri_factsheet_means_
to_african_amamerica.pdf. *Concise fact sheet explaining key provisions
of health care reform of specific interest to African Americans. Links to
other health care reform information can be found at* http://www.aarp
.org/health/health-care-reform/health_reform_factsheets.

United States Department of Health and Human Services. www.healthcare
.gov. *Comprehensive information on the health care reform law.*

ACKNOWLEDGMENTS

Writing this book has been one of the most challenging tasks I've ever undertaken . . . and one of the most rewarding. Not only have I shared knowledge in these pages, but I've learned so much about myself and my own health. First and foremost, I thank God. It was truly a leap of faith to dream and do this work. Many other people labored with me, and I am indebted to every one of them. I have to start by acknowledging my family. My husband, Derek, and my children, Kristin, James, and Justin, endured far too many days with me staring at a computer screen, physically present but otherwise disconnected from them and their activities. "Give me just a little more time," I'd ask them. And they graciously gave me a lot more time. I love you all. My mother, Gloria Abram, must be thanked, because by example she instilled in me the confidence to achieve anything I put my mind to do. I could never have conceived of writing a book without her. I also thank my sister, Donna Abram, for her eternal optimism, encouragement, and support. I am grateful to Donna Jacobs, who, although not in the publishing industry, was responsible for connecting me to Yale University Press through Liz Pelton. To Jean Thomson Black, the best executive editor ever, I thank you for your limitless patience, guidance, and encouragement. To Regina Brooks, a smart and relentless agent, thank you for believing in this book and for continually pushing me to make it better. Many thanks to Jaya Chatterjee and Laura Jones Dooley, who skillfully ushered my manuscript along and helped me better understand the publication process. I thank Tiffany Tate for reviewing the early (and not so good) chapters of this book; and I thank Stephanie Bailey and LaShawn McIver for reviewing the entire manuscript and offering honest feedback. Among the many other people to whom I'm grateful, I must thank Dr. Ben Carson and Dr. Georges Benjamin for offering their key endorsements of this work when it was nothing more than a proposal. Finally, to the dozens of friends, acquaintances, and strangers who offered so many words of encouragement to me along the way, please know that those words were just what I needed to see this book through to completion. May God bless you all.

INDEX

Page numbers in italics refer to illustrations.